Administrative Data and Child Welfare Research

Every day, social service agencies collect millions of pieces of data about the children and families they serve. Agencies depend on this data to inform decision-making by personnel throughout the organization and to provide meaningful research and evaluation on program effectiveness and outcomes. As capacity for collecting and utilizing data has increased so has the recognition that this data can and should be used more broadly. Further, it should include not just single-system data, but data across different human service agencies.

Administrative/big data systems can be powerful tools in increasing the efficiency and effectiveness of public child welfare services. Understanding, harnessing, and using big data holds tremendous promise in creating transformative change in the social services. Data analytics and data mining can lead to a better understanding of what services work for specific populations (targeting and predictive modelling), provide a more nuanced understanding of service outcomes for the workforce and major stakeholders (transparency), and facilitate collaboration across existing service delivery silos to reduce duplication of services and enhance consumer access to services (efficiency).

This book was originally published as a special issue of the *Journal of Public Child Welfare*.

Terry V. Shaw is Director of the Ruth H. Young Center for Families and Children and an Associate Professor in the School of Social Work at the University of Maryland, USA. His research is focused on the experience of children in the child serving systems and how to leverage existing administrative data systems to improve policy and practice.

Bethany R. Lee is the Associate Dean for Research and an Associate Professor in the School of Social Work at the University of Maryland, USA. Her research is centered on services for youth involved in the public systems of child welfare and/or mental health.

Jill L. Farrell is a Research Assistant Professor in the School of Social Work at the University of Maryland, USA. Her research centers on evidence-based practices and the use of data to inform policy, with particular regard to juvenile justice.

Administrative Data and Child Welfare Research

Using Linked Data to Improve Child Welfare Research, Policy, and Practice

Edited by
Terry V. Shaw, Bethany R. Lee and Jill L. Farrell

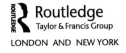

LONDON AND NEW YORK

First published 2018
by Routledge
2 Park Square, Milton Park, Abingdon, Oxon, OX14 4RN, UK

and by Routledge
711 Third Avenue, New York, NY 10017, USA

Routledge is an imprint of the Taylor & Francis Group, an informa business

British Library Cataloguing in Publication Data
A catalogue record for this book is available from the British Library

ISBN 13: 978-1-138-29592-6

Typeset in Minion
by RefineCatch Limited, Bungay, Suffolk

Publisher's Note
The publisher accepts responsibility for any inconsistencies that may have
arisen during the conversion of this book from journal articles to book chapters,
namely the possible inclusion of journal terminology.

Disclaimer
Every effort has been made to contact copyright holders for their permission to
reprint material in this book. The publishers would be grateful to hear from any
copyright holder who is not here acknowledged and will undertake to rectify
any errors or omissions in future editions of this book.

Contents

Citation Information

The chapters in this book were originally published in the *Journal of Public Child Welfare*, volume 10, issue 4 (September 2016). When citing this material, please use the original page numbering for each article, as follows:

Chapter 1
Four Principles of Big Data Practice for Effective Child Welfare Decision Making
Bridgette Lery, Jennifer M. Haight, and Lily Alpert
Journal of Public Child Welfare, volume 10, issue 4 (September 2016), pp. 466–474

Chapter 2
Child Well-Being: Where Is It in Our Data Systems?
Melissa Jonson-Reid and Brett Drake
Journal of Public Child Welfare, volume 10, issue 4 (September 2016), pp. 457–465

Chapter 3
Dual-System Families: Cash Assistance Sequences of Households Involved With Child Welfare
JiYoung Kang, Jennifer L. Romich, Jennifer L. Hook, JoAnn S. Lee, and Maureen Marcenko
Journal of Public Child Welfare, volume 10, issue 4 (September 2016), pp. 352–375

Chapter 4
Antipsychotic Use and Foster Care Placement Stability Among Youth With Attention-Deficit Hyperactivity/Disruptive Behavior Disorders
Ming-Hui Tai, Terry V. Shaw, and Susan dosReis
Journal of Public Child Welfare, volume 10, issue 4 (September 2016), pp. 376–390

Chapter 5
From Maltreatment to Delinquency: Service Trajectories After a First Intervention of Child Protection Services
Catherine Laurier, Sonia Hélie, Catherine Pineau-Villeneuve, and Marie-Noële Royer
Journal of Public Child Welfare, volume 10, issue 4 (September 2016), pp. 391–413

CITATION INFORMATION

Chapter 6

Children in Out-of-Home Care and Adult Labor-Market Attachment: A Swedish National Register Study

Torun Österberg, Björn Gustafsson, and Bo Vinnerljung

Journal of Public Child Welfare, volume 10, issue 4 (September 2016), pp. 414–433

Chapter 7

The Relationship Between Child Maltreatment, Intimate Partner Violence Exposure, and Academic Performance

Lisa R. Kiesel, Kristine N. Piescher, and Jeffrey L. Edleson

Journal of Public Child Welfare, volume 10, issue 4 (September 2016), pp. 434–456

For any permission-related enquiries please visit:
http://www.tandfonline.com/page/help/permissions

Notes on Contributors

Lily Alpert, PhD, is a Researcher at Chapin Hall at the University of Chicago, USA. Her work focuses on research evidence use by child welfare agency administrators and the development of interventions that promote the adoption and diffusion of longitudinal methods in child welfare performance measurement.

Susan dosReis is an Associate Professor in the Department of Pharmaceutical Health Services Research at the University of Maryland, USA. She researches psychotropic medication use among children and adolescents, examining disparities in psychotropic use by age, race, and foster care involvement, characterizing psychotropic treatment by combined use with psychotherapy for ADHD, and use of multiple psychotropic medications, and assessing longitudinal patterns in antipsychotic treatment for adults with schizophrenia.

Brett Drake is Professor of Social Work at the Brown School, Washington University, USA. He researches matters of child welfare with a focus on early intervention cases of child neglect as well as the connections between socio-environmental conditions and child neglect.

Jeffrey L. Edleson, PhD, is the Dean and Professor in the School of Social Work at the University of California, USA. His current research examines the impact of adult violence on children and how social systems respond to these children.

Jill L. Farrell is a Research Assistant Professor in the School of Social Work at the University of Maryland, USA. Her research centres on evidence-based practices and the use of data to inform policy, with particular regard to juvenile justice.

Björn Gustafsson is Senior Professor in the Department of Social Work, University of Gothenburg, Sweden and a Research Fellow at the Institute for the Study of Labor (IZA), Bonn, Germany. His research interests include social policy, social assistance, immigrant issues, poverty, the distribution of income, and China.

Jennifer M. Haight, MA, is a Senior Researcher at Chapin Hall at the University of Chicago, USA and a senior staff member of the Center for State Child Welfare Data. She has worked extensively with public and private child welfare agencies, helping them use administrative data to evaluate and structure continuous program improvements.

Sonia Hélie, PhD, is a Research Scientist with the Research and Expertise Center for Youth in Difficulty at the CIUSS Centre-Sud-de-l'Ile-de-Montreal and Affiliated Professor of Psychology at University of Quebec at Montreal and University of Montreal, Canada.

Jennifer L. Hook is Associate Professor of Sociology at the University of Southern California, USA. Her research areas include gender, family demography, inequality, work-family, social policy, child welfare, and comparative sociology.

Melissa Jonson-Reid is Ralph and Muriel Pumphrey Professor of Social Work at the Brown School, Washington University, USA. The major focus of her work is understanding how to improve the behavioral, educational, and health outcomes associated with childhood exposure to trauma, particularly abuse and neglect.

JiYoung Kang is a PhD candidate at the University of Washington School of Social Work, USA. Her research interest focuses on how social policy contexts influence individual life chances and outcomes, in particular, poverty, inequality, and family economic well-being cross-nationally and within U.S. contexts.

Lisa R. Kiesel, PhD, MSW, is an Assistant Professor in the School of Social Work at St. Catherine University, USA. Her research interests include clinical practice with children, adolescents, and families, child welfare and promotion of equal opportunity, and inclusion.

Catherine Laurier, PhD, is a Research Scientist with the Research and Expertise Center for Youth in Difficulty at the CIUSS Centre-Sud-de-l'Ile-de-Montreal and Affiliated Professor of Psychology at the University of Sherbrooke and in Criminology at the University of Montreal, Canada.

Bethany R. Lee is the Associate Dean for Research and an Associate Professor in the School of Social Work at the University of Maryland, USA. Her research is centered on services for youth involved in the public systems of child welfare and/or mental health.

JoAnn S. Lee is an Assistant Professor in the Department of Social Work at George Mason University, USA. She is researching how young adults come to be disconnected from social institutions, such as the family, school, and employment.

Bridgette Lery, MSW, PhD, is a Senior Analyst at the San Francisco Human Services Agency, USA. She uses administrative data for research, evaluation, and performance measurement of child welfare and other social programs.

Maureen Marcenko is the Cressey Endowed Professor at the University of Washington School of Social Work, USA. Her research interests include the well-being of vulnerable children and families with an emphasis on the development and testing of interventions within public child welfare and other public service systems.

Torun Österberg is an Associate Professor in the Department of Social Work, University of Gothenburg, Sweden. Her research interests include poverty, migration, segregation, labor market, income distribution, and social policy.

Kristine N. Piescher, PhD, is the Director of Research and Evaluation at the Center for Advanced Studies in Child Welfare at the University of Minnesota, USA. Her areas of interest include child welfare, child and family well-being, sibling and family interactions, and research methodology.

Catherine Pineau-Villeneuve, MSc, is a doctorate candidate in Criminology at the University of Montreal, Canada.

Jennifer L. Romich is an Associate Professor at the University of Washington School of Social Work, USA. She studies resources and economics in families, with a particular emphasis on low-income workers, household budgets, and families' interactions with public policy.

Marie-Noële Royer, MSc, is a Research Professional with the School of Criminology at the University of Montreal, Canada.

Terry V. Shaw is Director of the Ruth H. Young Center for Families and Children and an Associate Professor in the School of Social Work at the University of Maryland, USA. His research is focused on the experience of children in the child serving systems and how to leverage existing administrative data systems to improve policy and practice.

Ming-Hui Tai completed her PhD at the Department of Pharmaceutical Health Services Research at the University of Maryland, USA. Her research interests included analysis of antipsychotic and other psychotropic medication use among youth in foster care and evaluation of the integration of mental health services in pediatric primary care on child mental health outcomes.

Bo Vinnerljung is Professor of Social Work at Stockholm University, Sweden. Most of his research work concerns vulnerable children's development over time.

Introduction

Terry V. Shaw, Bethany R. Lee, and Jill L. Farrell

Administrative data systems can be powerful tools in increasing the efficiency and effectiveness of public child welfare services. Every day, child welfare and social service agencies collect millions of pieces of data about the children and families they serve. Agencies depend on these data to inform decision-making by personnel throughout the organization and to conduct meaningful research and evaluation on practice, policy, and program effectiveness. However, the information collected and maintained in a single system's administrative database is limited and cannot, in and of itself, provide a full view of children and families. Each child- and family-serving agency has a piece of the puzzle surrounding family and youth well-being, and without the ability to collaborate across systems the full mosaic is incomplete.

There is a popular name for cross-system data integration at the individual level for overall program and systemic improvement—Big Data. For most people the term "Big Data" brings to mind stories of data breaches (e.g., bank accounts getting hacked), threats to personal privacy (e.g., concerns over confidentiality), and unethical research (e.g., research done without consent or the oversight of an institutional review board). However, Big Data is at its essence the distillation of meaning from an array of diffuse data sources. This distillation has to encompass what is commonly referred to as the V's of Big Data. The first three of these V's were put forward by an IT analyst in 2001 and consist of "Volume" (the total amount of data collected across the various platforms), "Velocity" (the speed of data access and data collection), and "Variety" (the various types of data being accessed) (Laney, 2001). These three domains cover data access and the sheer size of the data process but do not speak to the accuracy of the data to meet the needs of an organization or structure. "Veracity" (accuracy of the data) is a fourth V that is essential to insure that the vast amount of data being collected from the various sources is accurate and timely (Gardner, 2013). Finally, a fifth V of big data should be considered, especially for work in the human services; that is "Value" (whether the data provides systemic, programmatic or individual value that is worth the expense) (Shaw, Farrell, & Kolivoski, 2016).

The graphic below attempts to show the relationship between the five V's of Big Data mentioned earlier. The core of any big data project must be accuracy (Veracity). If the data being utilized is not accurate, it does not matter how much there is, how varied it is, nor how quickly the data is collected or accessed

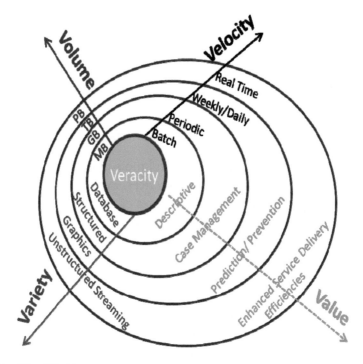

Figure 1: Five V's of Big Data
From *Shaw, Farrell, & Kolivoski, 2016.*

as there can be no real value. As the individual components expand (Volume, Velocity, and Variety) so does the potential Value that an agency might be able to glean from the data. Over time, the volume and velocity of data available to agencies has been increasing; however, the variety of data continues to be primarily coming from single agency data sources. This single system lens limits the amount of value or information available for decision-makers. In our opinion moving from the utilization of single system alone toward partnering with other child and family serving agencies is the key first step in moving toward Big Data.

But lost amid the buzzwords and catchphrases is what the concept of cross-system data integration (Big Data) can mean in the context of the human services. In essence, how can child- and family-serving agencies use the vast amount of information collected most efficiently, ethically, and effectively to better serve our populations and improve the overall efficiency of our practices, policies, and programs? How can we take Big Data and turn it into information that increases our understanding of the challenges and opportunities that exist to effectively serve children and families? Data collaboration done in a thoughtful and meaningful manner, in partnership with research professionals who are well versed in the statistical tools that are available, can help distill information from the various sources of data that will facilitate the ability to optimally serve children and families.

Understanding, harnessing, and using big data holds tremendous promise in creating transformative change in the social services. Data analytics and data mining can lead to a better understanding of what services work for specific populations (targeting and predictive modelling); provide a more nuanced understanding of service delivery and outcomes for the workforce and major stakeholders (transparency); and facilitate collaboration across existing service delivery silos to reduce duplication of efforts and allow for more efficient consumer access to services (efficiency). Innovative and important work aimed at encouraging agencies at the state, county, and local levels to collaborate is happening now, and these initiatives should be encouraged and expanded. A white paper published in partnership between the Substance Abuse Mental Health Services Association (SAMHSA) and the National Technical Assistance Center for Children's Behavioral Health discusses the concept of big data in the human services and how agencies can move from single system silos towards cross-system data collaboration (Shaw, Farrell, & Kolivoski, 2016). At the policy level, the Actionable Intelligence for Social Policy (AISP) initiative encourages data coordination through integrated data systems with the goal of facilitating policy and program innovation (AISP, 2016).

This text consists of methods, research, and discussions related to administrative or big data sets and their implications for the field of child welfare. The manuscripts collected here utilize multiple existing administrative data sets to provide cutting edge research that informs the field. Linking data across systems allows innovative questions to be empirically examined. For example, linking child welfare data with public assistance data allows for an examination of how public assistance might facilitate permanency (Kang, Romich, Hook, Lee, & Marcenko, chapter 3). For youth being treated with psychotropic medications, linking behavioral health and child welfare data allows the relationship between medication management and placement stability to be examined (Tai, Shaw, & dosReis, chapter 4). Child welfare involvement may also be predictive of future experiences with systems, including juvenile justice (Laurier, Hélie, Pineau-Villeneuve, & Royer, chapter 5) or even the labor workforce (Österberg, Gustafsson, & Vinnerljung, chapter 6). Another study examines academic performance among youth with experiences of maltreatment and/or intimate partner violence (Kiesel, Piescher, & Edleson, chapter 7). In addition to the empirical inquiries, we have included two commentaries related to the use of administrative data: one considers how well-being data could be integrated into child welfare administrative data (Jonson-Reid & Drake, chapter 2), and the other briefly summarizes four principles that underlie the effective use of administrative data by child welfare agencies for system improvement purposes (Lery, Haight, & Alpert, chapter 1).

The depth and breadth of information collected here is only available when agencies can move toward collaborative relationships with other public and private agencies to share data. It is our hope that this text will be illustrative of the significant and relevant findings that can be derived from research with big data in the human services. We also hope that it will provide systems with important considerations as they move forward with these initiatives, ideally with an eye toward moving away from single-system data analytic and casework practice, and toward a more integrated and collaborative process where data can be shared across child-serving systems.

References

Actionable Intelligence for Social Policy. (2016, June 7). Retrieved from http://www.aisp.upenn.edu/

Gardner, D. (February 22, 2013). The Open Group Panel Explores How the Big Data Era Now Challenges the IT Status Quo. The Open Group. http://blog.opengroup.org/tag/dana-gardner/

Jonson-Reid, M., & Drake, B. (2016). Child well-being: Where is it in our data systems? *Journal of Public Child Welfare, 10*(4), 457–465. DOI: 10.1080/15548732.2016.1155524

Kang, J., Romich, J. L., Hook, J. L., Lee, J. S., & Marcenko, M. (2016). Dual-system families: Cash assistance sequences of households involved with child welfare. *Journal of Public Child Welfare, 10*(4), 352–375.

Kiesel, L. R., Piescher, K. N., & Edleson, J. L. (2016). The relationship between child maltreatment, intimate partner violence exposure, and academic performance. *Journal of Public Child Welfare, 10*(4), 434–456.

Laney, D. "3D Data Management: Controlling Data Volume, Velocity and Variety". *Gartner.* 6 February 2001.

Laurier, C., Hélie, S., Pineau-Villeneuve, C., & Royer, M.-N. (2016). From maltreatment to delinquency: Service trajectories after a first intervention of child protection services. *Journal of Public Child Welfare, 10*(4), 391–413.

Lery, B., Haight, J. M., & Alpert, L. (2016). Four principles of Big Data practice for effective child welfare decision making. *Journal of Public Child Welfare, 10*(4), 466–474.

Österberg, T., Gustafsson, B., & Vinnerljung, B. (2016). Children in out-of-homecare and adult labor-market attachment: A Swedish National Register study. *Journal of Public Child Welfare, 10*(4), 414–433.

Shaw, T. V., Farrell, J., & Kolivoski, K. (2016). *Big data in human services* [Technical Brief]. Retrieved June 7, 2016, from National Technical Assistance Center for Children's Behavioral Health: http://files.ctctcdn.com/57c33206301/8d64082d-12e4-467d-b4dc-6f8c81f1ce71.pdf

Tai, M.-H., Shaw, T. V., & dosReis, S. (2016). Antipsychotic use and foster care placement stability among youth with attention-deficit hyperactivity/disruptive behavior disorders. *Journal of Public Child Welfare, 10*(4), 376–390.

Four Principles of Big Data Practice for Effective Child Welfare Decision Making

Bridgette Lery, Jennifer M. Haight, and Lily Alpert

ABSTRACT

Large administrative data systems are powerful tools that can aid child welfare decision making by allowing populations, trends, and risks to children to be described. But realizing the value that this "big data" can bring to improving the lives of children and their families requires one to (a) start the process by asking a question, (b) take a disciplined approach to converting data to evidence, (c) commit to the cyclical process of improvement using evidence, and (d) arrange and analyze the data in ways that maximize evidence yield. This article describes how these four principles can help agencies and researchers use big data wisely and in accordance with scientific standards as an instrument to generate evidence that fuels the cycle of continuous quality improvement.

Large administrative data systems are powerful tools that can aid decision making by allowing populations, trends, and risks to children to be described. But realizing the value that these "big data" can bring to improving the lives of children and their families requires adherence to four core principles:

1. The process of improvement starts with a question.
2. Converting data to evidence requires discipline.
3. The continuous quality improvement cycle demands evidence at each stage.
4. Certain techniques for arranging and analyzing big data can maximize evidence yield.

In this article, we describe knowledge and skills required to follow these principles. They have little to do with technical computer programming and more to do with pairing critical thinking with deep content knowledge. We argue that these skills should be taught to all staff, as all professional roles in a child welfare agency require critical thinking and would benefit from the use of evidence derived from big data to support good decision making. Regardless of the role of the consumers—be they agency staff, researchers, or advocates— without attention to these principles, big data may be underutilized or misused.

Principle 1: the process of improvement starts with a question

More and more, agencies, advocates, and other stakeholders are turning to analytic output to divine information that will help them improve their work. While the craving for information is, of course, the right intention, unless the desire for information is driven by the consumer's thoughtful question (one that can be answered with the available data), what may result is a somewhat passive relationship between the consumer and the data. Such a stance is common and understandable given how easy it is to produce reports, dashboards, and scorecards from big data. In addition, the flow of those documents is typically unidirectional from analysts or IT staff to leadership and managers. What this pattern doesn't account for is the role that the consumer must play by asking a specific question, the answer to which is needed to make a particular decision. In other words, the process of improvement does not in fact begin with access to information; rather, it begins with a question that we can use information sources to answer.

With that idea in mind, when approaching large administrative data sets as a source of information, it is important to remember that databases, no matter how large, in and of themselves, do not contain evidence. They simply contain *data*—bits and pieces of information about children and families that, while containing information on clients' characteristics and experiences, must be summarized in order to build a narrative about system performance. As obvious as that distinction may seem, clarity on this point is essential. Big data enable reliable summarization and the extraction of sturdy, representative patterns that can be used to guide system improvement, but getting there requires *analysis*. That analysis produces findings—that is, information that we might use as evidence to inform the claims, decisions, and actions that constitute improvement efforts. If the analysis is not conducted in accordance with scientific principles as described in the next section, the findings may not be interpretable as evidence of the claim, decision, or action they are intended to support.

The decision about which analytic method to employ depends on the question one wants to use the data to answer. Correctly matching the analysis to the question matters. For this reason, one of the axioms of administrative data analysis is the notion that *the process of improvement starts with a question* (Carnegie Foundation for the Advancement of Teaching, n.d.; Wulczyn, Alpert, Orlebeke, & Haight, 2014). The path from asking a research question to applying the findings is detailed in Figure 1.

Principle 2: converting data to evidence requires discipline

The value of big data is realized when large databases are subjected to analyses that answer thoughtful questions. As in any field, analysis has its own best practices, and in this case, those practices are derived from scientific standards

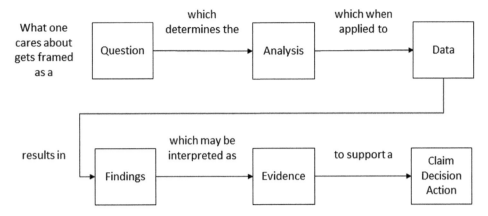

Figure 1. The process of improvement.

for measurement. For this reason, the second fundamental principle of big data analysis is that *converting data to evidence requires rigor—or what we call discipline*. Two critical elements of this discipline are (a) correctly identifying the risk set, also known as the study population or the denominator, and (b) aligning measurement of change over time with the period or window during which change is expected to occur.

The risk group

One principle of disciplined measurement is that when seeking to understand what is likely to happen in a child welfare system—whether the question is about trajectories through the system, the effectiveness of an intervention, or the dynamics of the workforce—one must select a population or *a denominator* that includes every subject who is at risk of experiencing the phenomena that one seeks to understand. For example, Figure 2 displays median duration in a foster care system for three populations that could be used to answer a question about how long children stay in care. The point-in-time and exit calculations are biased; the former examines only children still in care on the day in question and the latter examines only children who have left. The entry cohort analysis is the only one that captures the experience of all children moving through the system and, therefore, is the only measure of typical length of stay and changes in duration over time.

The importance of using an entry cohort to answer questions about likelihood, change over time, or what's typical for children in the system cannot be understated (Courtney, Needell, & Wulczyn, 2004). Though the child welfare field is more aware today than ever before of the biases inherent to exit and point-in-time analyses, methods that rely on exit and point-in-time cohorts are still widely used to make statements—often incorrect—about performance.

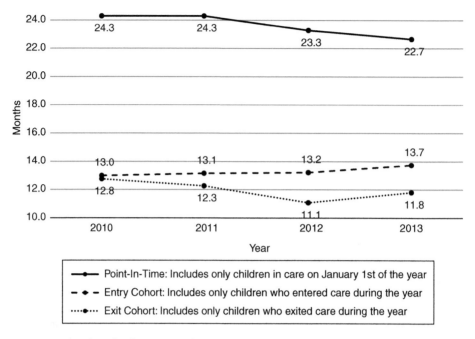

Figure 2. Median length of stay using three different denominators.

The window

The second element of disciplined measurement requires the measurement of change over time to be aligned with the period during which change is expected to occur. Well-designed administrative data files are extremely flexible, permitting an analyst to reorganize the records to support analysis that not only relies on the proper denominator but also looks for activity during a specified period.

Figure 3 helps illustrate this idea for a population of children in care on 1/1/2013 and observed for 2 years, through 1/1/2015. Suppose we are interested in reducing the likelihood of additional placement moves for children in

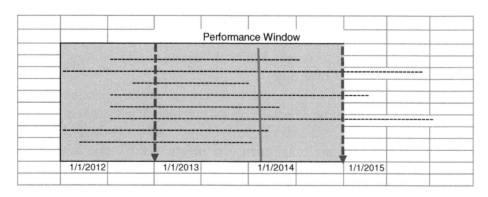

Figure 3. An in-care population in a 2-year window.

care on a given day. We know that children in this group will already have experienced some amount of movement and the goal of this intervention is to keep them from moving any *more*. To learn about the typical movement rate for an in-care population, we ask the question: Of all children who were in care on 1/1/2013, what proportion experienced at least one placement move in the *next 2 years*?

In the figure, the children in care are represented by the dashed horizontal lines. The window is contained within the dashed vertical lines. Moves that occurred prior to 1/1/2013 are not counted in the calculation. Why not? Because if we are trying to be predictive—that is, if we are trying to learn about the typical pattern of future instability so that we might prevent placement moves for a future group of children in care—then we must ask a question about what's *likely* to happen. We cannot change what has *already* happened, so we don't count moves that took place before the start of the window. When we set out to intervene with a future in-care population, we won't be able to change their prior moves, either; interventions can only affect what is yet to happen. By the same token, measuring placement moves for children admitted to care (as opposed to already in care) would also have to be measured prospectively. One would do this by examining an entry cohort of children and counting all of their moves, starting from their first day in care through to the end of the observation window.

Principle 3: the continuous quality improvement cycle demands evidence at each stage

In the child welfare field, the desire for evidence produced from administrative data has met a policy environment that has coalesced around the Continuous Quality Improvement (CQI) process. CQI is a cycle of problem-solving activities that requires the deliberate use of evidence at every stage (Wulczyn et al., 2014). Many different models exist that describe the process (Antony & Banuelas, 2002; Sokovic, Pavletic, & Kern Pipan, 2010), but all of them boil down to the same four fundamental phases: Plan, Do, Study, and Act (PDSA; O'Neill et al., 2011; Taylor et al., 2014). These stages put child welfare professionals through the paces of hypothesis development and testing— observe a problem, hypothesize as to why it exists, implement a potential solution, study whether that intervention had the desired effect, and make the next decision in response to those findings. The stages clarify that, while not always linear, the process of problem solving involves a sequence of activities that is important to follow.

When responsive to the first two principles, discussed above, administrative data analysis can and often should provide the evidence needed to support the claims, decisions, and actions inherent to the CQI process. For instance, consider a state child welfare agency that wants to increase the proportion of children exiting foster care to permanency within 12 months. Administrative data analysis can provide the evidence needed to define the problem ("Of children entering foster care during a given entry window, what proportion exit within 12 months and how does that outcome vary among subpopulations within my system?"). It may also provide insight into the drivers of variation ("I know that infants are more likely than older children to exit to adoption, which typically takes longer than reunification—does Acme County's admissions population have a large proportion of infants?"). Administrative data can also support the evaluation of selected interventions ("Has the likelihood of permanency within 12 months in Acme County increased since we started implementing Program X?"). Depending on the data the state collects, administrative data analysis may also be able to support a process evaluation ("Program X requires a caseload of eight children per worker and requires the worker to conduct a needs assessment every month— are those things happening?"). These are just a few examples. The point is that by identifying the junctures that are inherent to problem solving, CQI frameworks highlight that different types of evidence—often sourced in big data—are needed at different points in the process.

Principle 4: certain techniques for arranging and analyzing big data can maximize evidence yield

The final principle involves paying careful attention to the collection, configuration, and analysis of raw data in a way that maximizes its evidence-yielding potential and minimizes the possibility of getting the wrong answer. In this area, we offer four pieces of advice:

Be parsimonious. The availability of big data makes it alluring to mine the data rather than strategically narrow the search. It is tempting to add many variables to a model in the hopes of seeing what returns as statistically significant. However, given enough data, some factors will tend to reach significance, even though they may not be substantively meaningful or logically relevant (Rubin & Babbie, 2001). In short, when looking for predictors, if everything matters, nothing matters. The first principle of big data practice offers some protection against the temptation to engage in data mining by focusing on the information needed to answer a specific question and to identify levers for change.

Make the most of the data you have. Useful questions more naturally emerge from a well-designed database. Widening a database to augment it with more attributes about children or events can be desirable. However, sometimes the investment required (and the potential for incomplete data entry in those fields) contributes less value than simply making good use of the data already available in a "long" file. Additionally, a long file can consist of events that individuals experience over time. For instance, a long file that contains a "row" for each address change (as opposed to a row for each child) can produce information about children's residential mobility; a database that overwrites old addresses with the most recent ones cannot.

Look for variation that points to opportunities for change. Simply by observing variation, often with only a few variables, one can identify subpopulations at elevated risk for poor outcomes. For example, a great number of studies have identified variation in risk of foster care outcomes within a handful of subgroups (e.g., county, age, race/ethnicity, placement type) using California's child welfare administrative data (Courtney, 1994; Needell, Brookhart, & Lee, 2003; Shaw, 2006; Shlonsky, Webster, & Needell, 2003). The California Child Welfare Indicators Project, a publicly available online version of these data in simplified and aggregated format, allows administrators to identify differences in outcomes between these subgroups and use that evidence to design program improvements (State of California, California Department of Social Services, 2011; San Francisco Human Services Agency, 2015).

Use advanced methods when appropriate to improve precision. Outcomes for children involved in the child welfare system are not only influenced by individual and case-related factors but also by aspects of the environment in which they are served. When administrative data sets capture data on those contextual factors, certain analytic tools can account for those influences, further clarifying subpopulations that need attention. For instance, multilevel models (Raudenbush & Bryk, 2002) can reveal the effects of county characteristics, provider agencies, or regional socioeconomic dynamics on outcomes for children, independent of factors characterizing individual children (Wulczyn, Alpert, Martinez, & Weiss, 2015; Wulczyn, Gibbons, Snowden, & Lery, 2013). Long used in other aspects of social science, explicitly accounting for the role of ecological conditions using capable methods is still relatively new to child welfare.

It is noteworthy that the federal government has also endorsed this approach in its methodology for evaluating (and comparing) state agency performance in the third round of the Child and Family Service Review. These methods acknowledge the utility of multilevel models in accounting for the nested structure of child welfare administrative data, in this case, children nested within states (Administration for Children and Families, 2015), and for the fact that case mix and admission rates affect outcomes for children in foster care. A challenge for researchers is to translate findings derived from complex methods so they can be used by agency and advocate consumers.

Discussion

The goal of being driven by data misses the mark if it permits us to reflexively generate and consume information disconnected from a relevant question (Lery, Wiegmann, & Duerr Berrick, 2015). Such a dynamic removes consumers' agency in asking and answering questions germane to problem solving, as if the bits and bytes themselves can take the helm and steer change or improvement. Making the most out of administrative data or any other big data requires us to reframe our relationship with data into one that highlights the consumer's role—and responsibility—in generating necessary evidence needed to drive change. From that perspective, the principles of big data practice for child welfare decision making are in fact principles to guide professionals' own behavior. The data are merely the source of raw information, which are converted to evidence through the process of aligning good questions with the most relevant pieces of information, transformed using the right methods (Wulczyn et al., 2014). With these principles in mind and equipped with the skills necessary to uphold them, child welfare administrative data consumers should be ever aware that data yields its most valuable contribution when science—the disciplined process of asking and answering questions—produces knowledge that facilitates good decision making.

Acknowledgments

The authors are grateful to Britany Orlebeke and Fred Wulczyn at Chapin Hall at the University of Chicago for their feedback on drafts of this article, and for their thought leadership in the use of child welfare administrative data to improve children's lives.

References

Administration for Children and Families. (2015). *Child and family service review technical bulletin #8-amended*. Retrieved from https://training.cfsrportal.org/resources/3105#CFSR

Antony, J., & Banuelas, R. (2002). Key ingredients for the effective implementation of Six Sigma program. *Measuring Business Excellence*, 6(4), 20–27.

Carnegie Foundation for the Advancement of Teaching. (n.d.). *The six core principles of improvement*. Retrieved from http://www.carnegiefoundation.org/our-ideas/six-core-princi ples-improvement/

Courtney, M. (1994). Factors associated with the reunification of foster children with their families. *Social Service Review, 68*(1), 81–108.

Courtney, M., Needell, B., & Wulczyn, F. (2004). Unintended consequences of the push for accountability: The case of national child welfare performance standards. *Children and Youth Services Review, 26,* 1141–1154.

Lery, B., Wiegmann, W., & Duerr Berrick, J. (2015). Building an evidence-driven child welfare workforce: A university-agency partnership. *Journal of Social Work Education, 51*(Suppl. 2), S283–S298.

Needell, B., Brookhart, M. A., & Lee, S. (2003). Black children and foster care placement in California. *Children and Youth Services Review, 25*(5/6), 393–408.

O'Neill, S. M., Hempel, S., Lim, Y. W., Danz, M. S., Foy, R., Suttorp, M. J., et al. (2011). Identifying continuous quality improvement publications: What makes an improvement intervention "CQI"? *British Medical Journal Quality and Safety, 20,* 1011–1019.

Raudenbush, S. W., & Bryk, A. S. (2002). *Hierarchical linear models: Applications and data analysis methods* (2nd ed.). Newbury Park, CA: Sage.

Rubin, A., & Babbie, E. (2001). *Research methods for social work* (4th ed.). Belmont, CA: Wadsworth/Thompson Learning.

San Francisco Human Services Agency. (2015). *California child and family services review: Annual system improvement plan progress report, year 1.*

Shaw, T. (2006). Reentry into the foster care system after reunification. *Children and Youth Services Review, 28,* 1375–1390.

Shlonsky, A., Webster, D., & Needell, B. (2003). The ties that bind: A cross-sectional analysis of siblings in foster care. *Journal of Social Service Research, 29*(3), 27–52.

Sokovic, M., Pavletic, D., & Kern Pipan, K. (2010). Quality improvement methodologies—PDCA cycle, RADAR matrix, DMAIC and DFSS. *Journal of Achievements in Materials and Manufacturing Engineering, 43*(1), 476–483.

State of California, California Department of Social Services. (2011). *Program improvement plan for the child welfare services program*. Retrieved from http://www.childsworld.ca.gov/res/pdf/ PIP_Reformat_04_18_2011.pdf

Taylor, M. J., McNicholas, C., Nicolay, C., Darzi, A., Bell, D., & Reed, J. E. (2014). Systematic review of the application of the plan–do–study–act method to improve quality in healthcare. *BMJ Quality and Safety, 23*(4), 290–298.

Wulczyn, F., Alpert, L., Martinez, Z., & Weiss, A. (2015). *Within and between state variation in the use of congregate care*. Chicago, IL: Center for State Child Welfare Data, Chapin Hall at the University of Chicago.

Wulczyn, F., Alpert, L., Orlebeke, B., & Haight, J. (2014). *Principles, language, and shared meaning: Toward a common understanding of CQI in child welfare*. Chicago, IL: Center for State Child Welfare Data, Chapin Hall at the University of Chicago.

Wulczyn, F., Gibbons, R., Snowden, L., & Lery, B. (2013). Poverty, social disadvantage, and the black/white placement gap. *Children and Youth Services Review, 35*(1), 65–74.

Child Well-Being: Where Is It in Our Data Systems?

Melissa Jonson-Reid and Brett Drake

ABSTRACT

Child well-being is a required goal for public child welfare. Despite this requirement, there continues to be no systematic inclusion of child well-being indicators in administrative data, particularly for children remaining in the home. This brief commentary provides a rationale and suggested steps for moving toward inclusion of well-being indicators as a part of standard electronic record-keeping. Suggested operationalized elements for inclusion in electronic records are offered as well as suggestions for linkage across systems to begin to capture elements of the outcome of well-being automatically. Limitations and barriers are discussed as well as present policy changes that may provide support for this endeavor.

Since the 1980s child welfare has been charged with addressing child safety, preservation/reunification of the family, and permanency (Costin, Karger, & Stoesz, 1997). Data systems reflect this focus, describing reports of maltreatment, findings of investigations, services, and actions taken (U.S. Department of Health and Human Services [US DHHS], 2015). Substantial room for improvement exists, but core data elements exist nationally allowing monitoring of 1980s-era policy mandates. In 1997, The Adoptions and Safe Families Act (ASFA) included "well-being" as a focus of child welfare that was later operationalized by the Administration of Children and Families in the Child and Family Services Reviews (CSFRs) (Antle, Christensen, Van Zyl, & Barbee, 2012). The CFSRs included new items under the heading "Child and Family Well-Being Outcomes" to evaluate conformity with federal regulations (45 Code of Federal Regulations [CFR] Parts 1355, 1356, and 1357; US DHSS, n.d.). It would seem logical that the past two decades of emphasis on well-being would have brought about changes in state management information systems (MIS); however, this effect has not been the case. Such systems still remain almost totally blind to the issue of well-being. Bill Gates said "I am struck by how important measurement is to improving the human condition. You can achieve incredible progress if you set a clear goal and find a measure that will drive progress toward that goal" (2013). The application of this perspective to "well-being" in child welfare is clearly disquieting. Why has so little progress been made?

At least three barriers to the inclusion of well-being indicators exist in administrative data systems. The first relates to debate surrounding the operationalization of child well-being, ranging from the more concrete (Lanier, Kohl & Guo, 2015) to the philosophical (Raghavan & Alexandrova, 2015). The former definition might lead one toward adopting indicators like access to a medical home. A more philosophical or capacity development approach requires locating proxies indicative of a child's future potential. A second barrier may be a reticence to measure actions or outcomes not directly under the control of child welfare agencies (e.g., immunizations, mental health services, delinquent behavior) due to anxiety about being held responsible for availability of outside resources (Barth & Jonson-Reid, 2000). Finally, there is a concern that adding other measures simply adds more paperwork, which is already seen as a barrier to workforce retention (Ellett, Ellis, & Westbrook, 2007). The goal of this commentary is to discuss these barriers, offer a rationale for moving forward, and discuss opportunities and ideas for gradual integration of well-being into administrative data systems.

Next steps in recording child well-being

In regard to the first potential barrier, we do not assert that administrative data can capture all aspects of well-being. Nor do we believe that the CFSR child well-being outcomes and items measure capacity. CFSR requires the following outcomes to be demonstrated relative to well-being:

- Outcome 1: Families have enhanced capacity to provide for their children's needs —Needs and services of child, parents, and foster parents (Item 17), Child and family involvement in case planning (Item 18), Caseworker visits with child (Item 19) and Caseworker visits with parent(s) (Item 20).
- Outcome 2: Children receive appropriate services to meet their educational needs —Educational needs of the child (Item 21).
- Outcome 3 [Child and Family Well-Being]: Children receive adequate services to meet their physical and mental health needs—Physical health of the child (Item 22), Mental/behavioral health of the child (Item 23) (US DHHS, n.d.).

Clearly, these are general and process-oriented "measures" that are elements of setting the stage for well-being rather than realizing its achievement. In contrast, it is important to know if efforts are made to create the minimal contextual support needed to promote healthy development. In other words, a child's well-being whether measured in terms of a health outcome or internal capacity does not exist independent of external contextual factors that inhibit or aid positive development.

We therefore suggest considering child well-being as including two related parts, each of which is desirable as an end in its own right, including: *psychological/developmental well-being* or the degree to which a child develops capacities for success in the future and is emotionally and behaviorally sound (Raghavan & Alexandrova, 2015), and *contextual well-being*. Sullivan and Zyl (2008) remind us that well-being assumes a context which (a) provides the supports and conditions necessary to support adequate development of children in our society, and (b) protects a child's basic right to safety (Keenan, 2013). It is the recording of contextual well-being that we see as an incremental and important first step because it is consistent both with the CFSR and best practices in case management with multi-problem families, as well as a necessary if insufficient foundation for psychological and developmental well-being.

There are several issues to raise in regard to the organizational barriers related to concerns about misplaced accountability and worker burden. First, child welfare is primarily a case management system designed to assess needs and connect families and children to appropriate services to meet the goals of safety, permanency and well-being (Antle et al., 2012). Therefore referral and connection to outside resources are "usual care", at least for families who receive services beyond an investigation. Further, current systems innovations like differential response as well as the stated vision of the Children's Bureau to see child welfare embedded in an systems of care framework, suggest a continuing emphasis on this approach (Kyte, Trocme, & Chamberland, 2013; Mitchell et al., 2012).

Failing to effectively capture this process of moving from needs assessment, to service plan to outcomes in data systems creates at least three barriers to practice:

- increased burden in relation to response to CFSR;
- difficulty documenting innovations in practice like differential response or more structured approaches to case management; and
- barriers to continuity of care when worker turnover or transfer between programs occurs.

Lacking systematic collection of data that links needs, referrals and service engagement makes response to CFSR well-being outcomes reliant on case file reviews. Judgment of compliance is as dependent on record-keeping practices of a given worker as much as actual worker actions. Research suggests substantial variation in case recording practices (Huuskonen & Vakkari, 2015). To date, CFSR reviews have found the majority of states have been out of compliance with most well-being outcomes (Antle et al., 2012). It is impossible to know how much this is due a lack of worker action in the field versus incomplete case recording practices. Similarly, because innovations and evidence-based practices dependent on engaging families in case plans require an array of services to be identified and accessed, lack of systematic means of recording these efforts makes evaluation of outcomes dependent on case file review (Antle et al., 2012). Finally, there is a an argument to be made that lack of documentation of needs, services, and outcomes may help perpetuate gaps in resources increasing the risk that child welfare will be held liable for later untoward events that were outside the scope of CPS intervention.

While paperwork burden is oft cited as a reason for avoiding added data elements, this assumes a MIS system based on redundant and disconnected forms that are then subsequently uploaded into computers. A system designed to support case decision making rather than just report organizational level outcomes would potentially reduce, not increase "paperwork." Further, case management over time is often dependent on more than one worker due to transfers of responsibility as well as turnover. Effective and efficient services require continuity, which is often dependent on case records. Studies of reading of such records by workers have found that core information is hard to extract amidst the details spread out across documents over time (Huuskonen & Vakkari, 2015).

From here to there

While there are some indicators of needs and services present in the National Child Abuse and Neglect Data Systems (NCANDS) and Adoption and Foster Care Analyses and Reporting System (AFCARS), the fields are not well connected and many are commonly ignored. For example, an indicator of child disability has no relevant follow-up field indicating assessment for services or connection to services in health or education systems. Such data elements become a laundry list of items that may not at all be relevant to the case at hand and therefore more likely to be ignored (Gillingham, 2013). Nearly 20 years ago, Trocmé (1999) described a dilemma between data recording practices that were too qualitative and cumbersome for measurement of organizational outcomes and systems like the American State Automated Child Welfare Information Systems (SACWIS) that would be useful for management but have no utility for clinical case work decisions. This is not a necessary dichotomy. We agree with Gillingham (2013) that decisions about electronic systems cannot be made on outdated assumptions that were based on organizational responses rather than incorporating the needs of the frontline worker in executing effective practice. Both the advent of digital tools for recording and new approaches to developing relevant MIS systems have the potential to actually reduce paperwork and better support the well-being outcomes of children and families (Gillingham, 2013; Huuskonen & Vakkari, 2015).

As a place to start, we propose adding common-sense contextual well-being indicators that are consistent with the CFSR and prior research. These indicators reflect family capacity, child education, health and behavioral health. For example, completing primary and secondary educational milestones is a necessary step to achieving later productivity and capacity to enter the economic mainstream (Greenestone, Harris, Li, Looney & Patashnik, 2012; UNICEF, 2007). While completing educational milestones does not guarantee a state of well-being, it is a contextual requirement for facilitating future capacity. Ideally, indicators can apply across child ages by providing pull-down options that customize responses (e.g., referral to early childhood intervention compared to afterschool tutoring). Such indicators could be added as new fields within a system or obtained by automated linkage to other services. The brevity of this commentary precludes detailing data elements, but exemplars can be found in the 2014 Report on the Health and Well-being of Children (US DHHS, 2014), recommendations stemming from implementation of the Fostering Healthy Connections legislation (Deans et al., 2015), and other similar commentary (Sullivan & van Zyl, 2008).

After 18 years, why now?

We believe there is a unique combination of expectation of accountability, advances in technology and support for coordination between systems that provides a unique opportunity for bringing well-being to MIS table. We do not dwell on the increasing mandate for accountability here because it is evident in so many ways from the regular CFSR evaluations, to the expansion of lists of evidence-based practices (California Evidence-Based Clearinghouse for Child Welfare, n.d.), to the call for evidence-based approaches in funding mechanisms (Health Resources and Services Administration [HRSA], n.d.).

As mentioned earlier, services needed to meet a child's educational, health, and mental health needs are typically not provided by child welfare (Jonson-Reid, 2004; Freisthler, 2009). While avoidance of recording needs and services might seem somehow protective in regards to liability, we argue it may have the opposite effect. Criticisms of the CPS system inability to serve families abound —often based on assumptions that services are rejected or of poor quality (Jonson-Reid, 2011; Melton, 2005). The reality of the dependence of child welfare on external resources would be much easier to demonstrate if such information was systematically recorded. For example, a recent census study in Kentucky was able to identify regional gaps in services for youth in foster care (Sullivan & van Zyl, 2008). Such gaps are not something that can be "fixed" by better training of child welfare workers or lowered caseloads, this is a resource issue outside of child welfare. Such data need not be generated from isolated surveys alone, many communities are developing neighborhood indicator projects (Coulton & Korbin, 2007). Linkage of such indicators by geocoding addresses of clients would help map resource availability.

Second, there are windows of opportunity developing for data linkages required to meet the demands of policy. For children in foster care, there is federal legislation (Fostering Connections Act) requiring some type of coordination with health care providers (Jaudes et al., 2012). States like Texas have implemented a web-based health passport for youth in care in response to this policy (Mekonnen, Noonan & Rubin, 2009). Arguably such as system could be expanded to children receiving in-home services and tied into child welfare.

The genesis of funding for the creation of child welfare data systems came through federal support in the 1990s (Omnibus Budget Reconciliation Act of 1993—Public Law 103-66; PRWORA—Public Law 104-193). Title IV-E continues to provide some support for state and tribal agencies (45 CFR 1355.52). Newly proposed changes, if adopted, may make it easier for states to respond to the increasing demand for data linkages to other systems as well as changes to their own (45 CFR Part 95; Federal Register v 80, 154 proposed rules). The new proposed name for such systems is the *Comprehensive Child Welfare Information System (CCWIS)*. It is rare that movement in policy is so well aligned with practice demands.

Finally, criticisms of MIS and big data ideas are often grounded in the past. Increasingly we see demonstrations in the literature of how cross-system administrative data provide clear indicators of positive or negative functioning (Putnam-Hornstein, 2011; Jonson-Reid, Kohl, Drake, 2012). There are examples of such data systems being used to improve educational outcomes (Florida PK20 Education Data Warehouse, n.d.) and inform state policy and health services (Lee, Whitcomb, Galbreth & Patterson, 2010). Gillingham (2013) points out that substantial advances have been made in the design of electronic systems to meet the needs of caseworkers and interface preferences. Huuskonen and Vakkari (2015) remind us that the advent of inexpensive electronic data collection alternative such as handheld tablets can replace the need for duplicative structured forms and prevent problems due to readability of hand written notes. As technology and data security advances are made it is increasingly possible to query other systems for specific items like whether or not immunizations have been completed.

Conclusion

An obvious criticism of this discussion is that current systems focus on negative outcomes (e.g., whether or not a child commits a delinquent act or is treated for assault in the emergency room) limiting our ability to use system data to track well-being. Positive indicators, however, also exist (e.g., graduating from high school, educational proficiency test scores, post-secondary training, entering the workforce, owning a home). Eventually it may be possible to integrate more subjective measures of well-being into case records to examine real time evidence of functioning and better inform our ability to support a child's capacity (Ben-Arieh, 2008). Until that time, however, we believe that integrating contextual well-being as fields in MIS is key, timely, and will improve accountability to policy as well as benefit child welfare practice. We have a moral responsibility to assure that we are using every advantage technology can confer to improve the lives of children who come to the attention of CPS for maltreatment.

References

Adoptions and Safe Families Act of 1997 (H.R. 867) Public Law 105-89.

Antle, B. F., Christensen, D. N., Van Zyl, M. A., & Barbee, A. P. (2012). The impact of the solution-based casework (SBC) practice model on federal outcomes in public child welfare. *Child Abuse & Neglect, 36*(4), 342–353.

Barth, R. P., & Jonson-Reid, M. (2000). Outcomes after child welfare services: Implications for the financing and design of child welfare services. *Children and Youth Services Review, 22*(9/10), 787–810.

Ben-Arieh, A. (2008). The child indicators movement: Past, present, and future. *Child Indicators Research, 1*(1), 3–16.

California Evidence-Based Clearinghouse for Child Welfare. (n.d.). Website. http://www.cebc4cw.org/

Code of Federal Regulations [CFR] Title 45 Parts 1355, 1356, and 1357 Title IV–E Foster Care Eligibility Reviews and Child and Family Services State Plan Reviews. (2000, January). *Federal Register 65*(16).

Code of Federal Regulations [CFR] Title 45, Part 95; Proposed rules. (2014, October). *Federal Register, 80* (154).

Code of Federal Regulations [CFR] Title 45, Part 1355. Conditions for approval of funding. (1993, December). *Federal Register, 58* 67945, as amended at 77 FR 933, January 6, 2012.

Costin, L. B., Karger, H. J., & Stoesz, D. (1997). *The politics of child abuse in America.* Oxford, UK: Oxford University Press.

Coulton, C. J., & Korbin, J. E. (2007). Indicators of child well-being through a neighborhood lens. *Social Indicators Research, 84*(3), 349–361.

Deans, K. J., Minneci, P. C., Nacion, K. M., Thackeray, J. D., Scholle, S. H., & Kelleher, K. J. (2015). A framework for developing healthcare quality measures for children and youth in foster care. *Children and Youth Services Review, 58*, 146–152.

Ellett, A. J., Ellis, J. I., & Westbrook, T. M. (2007). A qualitative study of 369 child welfare professionals' perspectives about factors contributing to employee retention and turnover. *Children and Youth Services Review, 29*(2), 264–281.

Florida PK20 Education Data Warehouse. (n.d.). Website. http://edwapp.doe.state.fl.us/edw_facts.htm

Freisthler, B. (2009). *Need for and access to supportive services in the child welfare system: An analysis using geographic information systems (GIS)* [CCPR-037-09]. California, LA: UCLA, California Center for Population Research.

Gates, B. (2013, January). Bill Gates: My plan to fix the world's biggest problems. *Wall Street Journal.* Retrieved from http://www.wsj.com/articles/SB10001424127887323539804578261780648285 77

Gillingham, P. (2013). The development of electronic information systems for the future: Practitioners, "embodied structures" and "technologies-in-practice." *British Journal of Social Work*, *43*(3), 430–445.

Greenestone, M., Harris, M., Li, K., Looney, A., & Patashnik, J. (2012). *A dozen economic facts about K-12 education: The Hamilton Project*. Washington, DC: Brookings Institute.

Health Resources and Services Administration (HRSA). (n.d.). *The maternal, infant, and early childhood home visiting program partnering with parents to help children succeed*. Washington, DC: US DHHS. Retrieved from http://mchb.hrsa.gov/programs/homevisiting/programbrief.pdf

Huuskonen, S., & Vakkari, P. (2015). Selective clients' trajectories in case files: Filtering out information in the recording process in child protection. *British Journal of Social Work*, *45*(3), 792–808.

Jaudes, P. K., Champagne, V., Harden, A., Masterson, J., & Bilaver, L. A. (2012). Expanded medical home model works for children in foster care. *Child Welfare*, *91*(1), 9–33.

Jonson-Reid, M. (2004). Child welfare services and delinquency: The need to know more. *Child Welfare*, *83*(2), 157–174.

Jonson-Reid, M. (2011). Disentangling system contact and services: A key pathway to evidence-based children's policy. *Children and Youth Services Review*, *33*, 598–604.

Jonson-Reid, M., Kohl, P. L., & Drake, B. (2012). Child and adult outcomes of chronic child maltreatment. *Pediatrics*, *129*(5), 839–845.

Keenan, W. J. (2013). Children's rights and community well-being. *Pediatrics*, *131*(1), 3–4.

Kyte, A., Trocme, N., & Chamberland, C. (2013). Evaluating where we're at with differential response. *Child Abuse & Neglect*, *37*(2), 125–132.

Lanier, P., Kohl, P., & Guo, S. (2015, January). *Comparing child and caregiver assessments of child well-being in a sample of maltreated children*. Paper presented at Society for Social Work Research Annual Conference.

Lee, L., Whitcomb, K., Galbreth, M., & Patterson, D. (2010). A strong state role in HIE: Lessons from the South Carolina Health Information Exchange. *Journal of AHIMA*, *81*, 46–50.

Mekonnen, R., Noonan, K., & Rubin, D. (2009). Achieving better health care outcomes for children in foster care. *Pediatric Clinics of North America*, *56*(2), 405–415.

Melton, G. B. (2005). Mandated reporting: A policy without reason. *Child Abuse & Neglect*, *29*(1), 9–18.

Mitchell, L., Walters, R., Thomas, M. L., Denniston, J., McIntosh, H., & Brodowski, M. (2012). The Children's Bureau's vision for the future of child welfare. *Journal of Public Child Welfare*, *6*(4), 550–567.

Omnibus Budget Reconciliation Act of 1993. Public Law 103–66.

Personal Responsibility and Work Opportunity Reconciliation Act of 1996 (PRWORA). Public Law 104-193.

Putnam-Hornstein, E. (2011). Report of maltreatment as a risk factor for injury death: A prospective birth cohort study. *Child Maltreatment*, *16*, 163–174.

Raghavan, R., & Alexandrova, A. (2015). Toward a theory of child well-being. *Social Indicators Research*, *121*(3), 887–902.

Sullivan, D. J., & van Zyl, M. A. (2008). The well-being of children in foster care: Exploring physical and mental health needs. *Children and Youth Services Review*, *30*(7), 774–786.

Trocmé, N. (1999). Canadian child welfare multi-dimensional outcomes framework and incremental measurement development strategy. *Roundtable*. 30. Retrieved from http://cwrp.ca/sites/default/files/publications/en/RoundtableOutcomes.pdf#page=32

UNICEF. (2007). *Child poverty in perspective: An overview of child well-being in rich countries. Innocenti Report Card 7*. Florence, Italy: Innocenti Research Centre.

U.S. Department of Health and Human Services (US DHHS), Health Resources and Services Administration, Maternal and Child Health Bureau. (2015). *Child Maltreatment 2013*. Rockville, MD: Author.

U.S. Department of Health and Human Services (US DHHS), Health Resources and Services Administration, Maternal and Child Health Bureau. (2014). *The health and well-being of children: A portrait of states and the nation, 2011–2012.* Rockville, MD: Author.

U.S. Department of Health and Human Services (US DHHS), Health Resources and Services Administration, Maternal and Child Health Bureau. (n.d.). Child & Family Services Reviews. Retrieved from http://www.acf.hhs.gov/programs/cb/monitoring/child-family-services-reviews

Dual-System Families: Cash Assistance Sequences of Households Involved With Child Welfare

JiYoung Kang, Jennifer L. Romich, Jennifer L. Hook, JoAnn S. Lee, and Maureen Marcenko

ABSTRACT

Dual-system families, those involved with the child welfare system and receiving public cash assistance, may be more vulnerable than families connected to only one of the two systems. This study advances our understanding of the heterogeneous and dynamic cash-assistance histories of dual-system families in the post–welfare reform era. With merged administrative data from Washington over the period 1998–2009, we use cluster analysis to group month-to-month sequences of cash-assistance use among households over the 37-month period surrounding child removal. Close to two thirds of families who received any assistance either had a short spell with Temporary Assistance for Needy Families (TANF) or lost TANF. Smaller percentages had steady support. Families who lose assistance are less likely than average to reunify while those who connect to benefits are more likely, suggesting that coordination between systems may serve dual-system families well.

Child welfare caseloads disproportionally comprise poor families. Poverty is associated with child neglect (Connell-Carrick, 2003), child welfare referrals (Slack, Lee, & Berger, 2007), and child welfare involvement (Paxson & Waldfogel, 2002; Rivausx et al., 2008; Slack, 1999). In Washington state, over half of primary caregivers with children in out-of-home care report household incomes of less than $10,000 per year (Marcenko, Hook, Romich, & Lee, 2012). Some poor families draw support from public cash assistance; when these families are also child welfare–involved they are subject to the requirements of both systems. Major reforms to public assistance in the late 1990s resurfaced some long-standing questions about how well the cash assistance and child welfare systems serve their mutual clients and raised new concerns as well (Berrick, 1999, Frame, 1999). The 1996 replacement of Aid to Families With Dependent Children (AFDC) with Temporary Assistance for Needy Families (TANF) eliminated entitlement cash assistance in favor of time-limited support with tougher sanctions for noncompliance with program rules and strong work enforcement—all of which

Color versions of one or more of the figures in the article can be found online at www.tandfonline.com/wpcw.

were potentially difficult for dual-system families to reconcile with the demands of the child welfare system (Geen, Fender, Leos-Urbel, Markowitz, & the Urban Institute, 2001; McGowan & Walsh, 2000; Ward Doran & Roberts, 2002). At the same time, TANF also opened the possibility of greater collaborative efforts between welfare and child welfare agencies and offered states greater flexibility for dual-system families (Ehrle, Scarcella, & Geen, 2004).

In this article we document one facet of the intersection of child welfare and cash assistance in the post-reform era by examining cash-assistance benefits received by households from which a child is placed out-of-home. Drawing on a unique data set of administrative records for families with children removed from the home in Washington between 1999 and 2008, we describe patterns in the benefit-use sequences of dual-system families. Our aim is descriptive; we do not attempt to draw causal links between events. Rather our data and methods allow us to show the diversity of trajectories, documenting how child welfare households receive cash assistance in the post–welfare reform era.

Background

The substantial overlap between child welfare and welfare caseloads—TANF and its predecessor AFDC—is well documented (Courtney, Dworsky, Piliavin, & Zinn, 2005; Pelton 1989; Shook Slack, Holl, Lee, McDaniel, Altenbernd, & Stevens, 2003; U.S. Department of Health and Human Services, 2000; Waldfogel, 2004). Dual-system families may be more vulnerable than families connected to only one of two systems. They are more likely to have material hardships that may impede reunification than those families involved only in the child welfare system. They are also likely to experience more-demanding requirements from two different systems relative to families who participate in welfare programs only (Ward Doran & Roberts, 2002; Geen et al., 2001). Welfare and child welfare administrators and caseworkers report that dual-system families find the requirements of the two systems overwhelming (Geen et al., 2001). Whereas the cash welfare system encourages paid employment for mothers, the child welfare system puts the greatest emphasis on parents safely caring for children. Insofar as clashes between the demands of market work and caregiving create greater instability or inadequacy in resources for vulnerable families, this fundamental system-level conflict raises both pragmatic and moral considerations. Do stringent cash-assistance requirements reduce the chances of reunification, the preferred outcome of the child welfare system? In doing so, do they exacerbate hardship and suffering?

Poor families involved with the child welfare system can draw economic support from TANF, Supplemental Security Income (SSI), or General Assistance (GA) (Pecora, Whittaker, Maluccio, Barth, & Plotnick, 2009). Here we describe each of these programs, then turn to reasons why families might move on, off, or between these programs. Washington made changes to its TANF and GA programs after the observation period covered in this study, including a change that makes it more likely that a caregiver will retain TANF benefits after a child is removed from the home. We will consider possible implications of these more recent changes—and the discontinuity in the child welfare data that prevents us from examining them in the current analysis—in the discussion.

TANF serves as the primary monthly cash-assistance program for poor families, in particular, working-age adults with dependent children. Formed by the Personal Responsibility and Work Opportunity Reconciliation Act of 1996 (PRWORA), TANF provides cash grants and other assistance, conditioned on participating in work-related activities (e.g., career readiness training or supervised job search) for 30 hours per week in most cases. TANF policies vary from state to state; a comparison of state TANF programs shows that Washington state's policies were relatively generous in benefits and lenient in application of sanctions during the post–welfare era (Meyers, Gornick, & Peck, 2001). For instance, the state did not have a family cap, meaning that benefits would increase when an additional child was added to the family through birth or other means.

Supplemental Security Income supports poor families that contain an adult or child with a disability. In 2014, 4.6 million persons under age 65 received SSI (U.S. Social Security Administration, 2014). There is documented overlap between SSI and TANF recipients; 16.1% of TANF families are estimated to also include an SSI recipient (Wamhoff & Wiseman, 2006). Welfare reform may have increased SSI caseloads by providing incentives for individual families to move from TANF to SSI (Schmidt & Sevak, 2004) because it offers a higher monthly benefit without time limits or work requirements (Wamhoff & Wiseman, 2006). Fiscal constraints may have also produced political incentives for some states to turn to SSI because SSI grants are federally funded.

Third, during the time period covered by our data, some 30 states, including Washington state, also had GA programs that support those who qualify for neither TANF nor SSI. As a state or local program, GA program eligibility, benefit levels, and time limits vary across localities. Recipients are typically childless adults, including parents without minor children in the household. GA monthly grants are modest—lower than TANF grants and typically no more than $400 per month. Many programs have been cut or eliminated during the recent economic downturn (Schott & Cho, 2011). Seven states impose time limits for anyone receiving benefits, but their policies vary from a 1-year lifetime limit to an intermittent time limit such as 12 out of the last 60 months as of year 2015 (Schott & Hill, 2015). Washington state did not have a GA time limit during the study period.

Transitions of cash assistance use and their potential consequences

There are several likely transition sequences within and between the three cash-assistance programs for dual-system families. Child welfare involvement may initiate particular moves between, on to, or off of programs, and program eligibility may change when a child is placed out of the household.

As TANF is a primary source of public assistance and its use is typically conditional upon having a child in the household, we expect that some households will lose TANF after removal of a child. PRWORA provided an option for TANF benefits to continue if a child's absence was likely to be temporary (45 days or less), allowing states flexibility to some extent (Committee on Ways and Means, U.S. House of Representatives, 1996), but whether and how often this option was invoked in practice seems to be unknown. As we note in the discussion, Washington recently took advantage of later federal legislation to expand this temporary absence policy.

Even if benefits are not ceased upon child removal, TANF loss can also result from competing mandates from the conflicting philosophies between the two systems (McGowan & Walsh, 2000; Ward Doran & Roberts, 2002). For example, parents may experience conflicts when child welfare requirements (such as meetings, court attendance, and service participation) overlap with completing TANF job training or job search requirements. Parents might have to make choices between visitation with their children, scheduled at the convenience of the child welfare workers, and showing up for a job interview or pre-employment test, scheduled at the convenience of a potential employer. We expect that post-removal transitions off of TANF are likely to produce more economic hardships for dual-system families as they lose primary benefits, potentially creating a slow reunification outcome.

Other life circumstances could cause both a removal and TANF loss. For instance, a physical or mental health crisis could render a caregiver both unable to safely care for children and unable to comply with TANF requirements. In this case, a sequence of child removal would not cause the subsequent TANF loss; rather, both events would be consequences of another factor.

TANF loss may precede child removal. Evidence suggests that losing TANF is associated with child welfare involvement and may worsen child-protection outcomes. For instance, Shook Slack and colleagues (2007) examine families who received TANF in Illinois in 1999 and find that those whose income was cut due to a sanction for noncompliance with welfare rules were more likely to have been reported to Child Protective Services for reasons of neglect. One explanation for this sequence is that income loss destabilized the family leading to removal; however, as before, other factors could account for both TANF loss and child removal.

Child removal could result in other transitions—or not affect benefit use at all. Among all parents who lose TANF, in some cases, a parent from whom a child is removed may no longer meet the TANF requirements but could meet requirements for GA or SSI. Families who transit from TANF to these other cash-assistance programs may be better off than those losing benefits altogether or losing TANF. Transition to other cash assistance could yield different consequences. Movement from TANF to GA are likely to worsen families' economic status because benefit amounts are likely to reduce, while families transitioning from TANF to SSI may fare better because SSI grants are typically larger. SSI grants follow individuals, so grants to parents with disabilities would be unaffected by removal but if a recipient child leaves the household, the parent would no longer receive the grant.

Lastly, parents who come to the attention of the child welfare system may connect to TANF or other benefits. PRWORA provided states with greater flexibility in how they delivered services to poor families, which may have led state child welfare and cash-assistance systems to collaborate in order to better serve families on their mutual caseloads (Ehrle, Scarcella & Geen, 2004). In the event that child welfare workers determined that families needed additional income support, these collaborative efforts could have facilitated families gaining TANF, GA, or SSI after coming to the attention of the child welfare system.

We hypothesize that all of these patterns may be observed to some extent within the population. Hence our primary goal is to establish a set of types of sequences, or sequential patterns, that describe benefit use among families before and after a child is removed from the household. For instance, we suspect that families who have TANF until removal and then lose it may constitute one type of sequence. We use a data-driven–cluster-analysis approach to group sequences of benefit use over time in order to reveal patterns not a priori predicted. Having established a set of benefit sequence groups, we then address a set of research questions about the timing and correlates of benefit use. First, within these groups, to what extent do households maintain, gain, or lose benefits before, during, or after the period of child removal (Question 1)? Second, how do demographic and case characteristics relate to different benefit sequence groups (Question 2)? Third, how are benefit sequence groups associated with reunification outcomes (Question 3)? The data set, which applies to child welfare cases in which a child was removed from the caregiver's home, provides insight into the public financial support of families of greatest concern, those for whom abuse or neglect was substantiated as severe enough to warrant removal.

This study adds to the knowledge base in important ways. Previous studies examining benefit use among dual-system families focus on AFDC and TANF (Slack, 1999; Wells & Guo, 2003, 2004, 2006; Kortenkamp, Geen, & Stagner, 2004). Our analysis includes SSI, which is an increasingly important support for poor families, and GA, which was an important source of support in the 2000s and the most common state-administered type of grant for adults without children in the household. Extant work also uses dichotomous measures of welfare continuity (versus loss) or uses counts of months on benefits to measure continuity. We use a more flexible, empirical approach that allows us to examine transitions on to and off of three different types of cash assistance (TANF, SSI, and GA) and combinations thereof. Finally, by relying on administrative data with a large number of observations and an analytic approach that clusters cases by the sequence of benefits used and not used, we can reveal both common and less common patterns including those not a priori considered.

Method

Case universe and data

This study uses child welfare and public assistance data from the Washington State Health Service Department (HSD) and was conducted with approval from the Washington State Institutional Review Board. Figure 1 summarizes the process by which we assembled the data set capturing the population of dual-system families in this state. First, using child welfare records we identified primary caregivers whose child was removed for the first time from July 1999 through May 2008 (for details, see Hook, Romich, Lee, Marcenko, & Kang, 2016). Primary caregivers are typically parents and most commonly mothers. In Washington state, child removals happen when child-protection investigators substantiate imminent risk of abuse or neglect and also in the case of child behavioral issues requiring institutional care.[1] The first date of removal was used to include only one record per caregiver. Caregivers 18 or older and younger than 65 were included, as persons outside this age range would be eligible for Social Security and other supports. This yielded 26,806 caregivers, the universe of cases meeting the above parameters.

Cases included in our analysis reflect the demographics of the Washington state child welfare caseload during this time period. Primary caregivers are most commonly women (88.2%) and on average are 33.3 years old when their children are removed. The largest percentage identify as non-Hispanic White (70.0%) followed by Hispanic (8.5%), Native American (8.3%), African American (7.7%), Asian/Pacific Islander (2.2%), and others (3.3%). Non-exclusive reasons for removals reported are neglect (47.0%), substance abuse (23.5%), physical abuse (16.7%), and sexual abuse (4.9%). More than two thirds of the cases (68.3%) had more than two reasons for removal indicated. In more than two thirds of our study cases (67.6%) children were reunited with their caregivers within 18 months of removal. Among reunifying families, the average time between removal and reunification was 116.5 days.

Lastly, we match 26,806 primary-caregiver cases to cash-assistance data for January 1998 through December 2009 in the Washington State Human Services Department (HSD). This finds that a total of 16,556 households (61.8% of the universe, Figure 1) received cash assistance for at least 1 month during the observation period of 37 months, which consists of 18 months prior to the removal month, the month of removal, and 18 months after removal. We used the same approach as Wells and Guo (2003) in setting the observation window to focus on benefit-use experiences of child welfare–involved families around child removal. As such, the chronological time associated with the observation

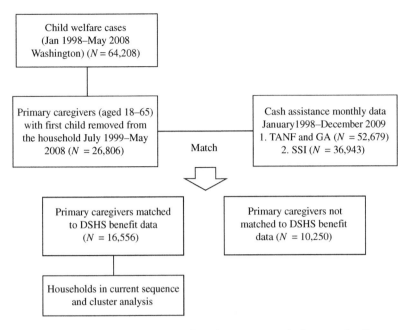

Figure 1. Data set construction for universe of Washington state dual-system families.

window is case specific. For example, for a household from which a child was removed in July 2005, the data would contain cash-assistance records from January 2004 through to January 2008, a total of 37 months. Our data contain the TANF cash assistance received by the caregiver. This could be either a family or child-only grant. This would not include a child-only grant where someone other than the caregiver was the payee (i.e. foster parent).

Analysis

Because households involved with the child welfare system likely include a heterogeneous mix of different benefit-use patterns, our approach is to characterize sequences and then create groups, or clusters, of similar sequences. We construct sequence data for the 16,556 households who received cash assistance during the period starting 18 months before the month of child removal and extending 18 months after, for a total of 37 months. Eight states of benefit participation status are possible each month: (1) TANF, (2) SSI, (3) GA, (4) TANF + SSI, (5) TANF + GA, (6) SSI + GA, (7) TANF + SSI, GA, or (8) no public income benefits. Hence the sequence for each primary caregiver consists of the ordered listing of these states for the 37-month observation period. Sequence analysis treats sequence data; that is, all of the listed successive (sequential) elements in a series of events, as a whole entity rather than discrete events (Abbott & Hrycak, 1990; Aisenbrey & Fasang, 2010; Brzinsky-Fay, Kohler, & Luniak, 2006; Gabadinho, Ritschard, Studer, & Nicolas, 2010), focusing on a holistic trajectory of "events in context" instead of "entities with variable attributes" (Aisenbrey & Fasang, 2010, p. 422).

We use the optimal matching (OM), the most commonly used sequence dissimilarity measure to gauge resemblance between sequences. The OM algorithm calculates the overall distance between two sequences by counting the number of substitutions, insertions, and deletions (indels) needed to make two sequences the same (for details, see Abbott & Hrycak, 1990) and by adding these to the respective costs, referred to as the Levenshtein distance (Aisenbrey & Fasang, 2010; Brzinsky-Fay et al., 2006). This process finds the most efficient way (minimum distance) to switch from one sequence to another sequence. The substitution cost is concerned with the timing of states; that is, whether the same state occurs at the same time point in two sequences. The indel cost captures the occurrence of states. We compute pairwise OM distances between sequences with an insertion/deletion cost of 1 and a substitution cost of 2, following Brzinsky-Fay (2007).

The distances measured by OM are used for cluster analysis in grouping similar sequences. In fact, a sequence analysis is often used in combination with a process of simplifying sequences such as cluster analysis. Despite the subjectivity of cluster analysis (Halpin & Chan, 1998; Piccarreta & Lior, 2010), this approach is by far the most popular method for identifying different subsets of sequences (Brzinsky-Fay et al., 2006; Havlicek, 2010; Pollock, 2014; Simonson, Gordo, & Titova, 2011). We employed hierarchical clustering with Ward linkage. Because conventional fit test statistics do not apply to cluster analysis with sequence data (Brzinsky-Fay, 2007; Pollock, 2014), our approach to choosing a number of groups is necessarily more qualitative. We consulted the clustering dendrogram, examined case counts, and analyzed descriptive statistics to determine how many groups are analytically meaningful. We then assigned names based on the dominant patterns within each group.

Results

Assistance receipt by benefit sequence group

The cluster analysis yielded six clusters, corresponding to sequence groups, displayed in Table 1. Here we briefly introduce each group by its major defining characteristics before presenting more-detailed information on monthly benefit participation rates and sequences below. Households with *Short Spells of TANF*, with only 7 months of average duration out of 37 months of observation in TANF use, constitute the largest group, with about a quarter of all households experiencing removal (25.2%) and 40.7% of households that ever used any cash assistance. *Lose TANF*, the second-most-frequent group, consists of households that were on TANF at the beginning of the observation but lost their benefits over time, especially around their child removal. They make up 15.7% of all households or about a quarter of benefit users (25%). Next is the *Gain Benefits* group, which gradually obtains GA, SSI,

Table 1. Clusters of benefit sequences.

Sequence cluster type	Number	Percentage of households using cash assistance	Percentage of all households
Short Spells of TANF	6,749	40.8	25.2
Lose TANF	4,201	25.3	15.7
Gain Benefits	1,905	11.5	7.1
Steady TANF	1,547	9.4	5.8
Steady SSI	1,255	7.6	4.7
TANF + SSI	899	5.4	3.4
No Assistance	10,250		38.2
Total	26,806	100	100

or TANF and remain on for most of the remainder of the observation period; 7.1% of households transitioned onto benefits during the observation period. This is about one in nine (11.5%) of all households who ever used benefits. Smaller numbers of households can be characterized as in the *Steady TANF* group (5.8% of all households), maintaining their TANF benefits for average of 31 months; *Steady SSI* (4.7%), who are on SSI average 26 months; or TANF + SSI, who began with the combination of TANF and SSI in the observation (3.4%). Next we describe the differences between groups, which confirm our expectation of heterogeneity of cash-assistance use trajectories.

Data for each group are displayed with benefit states aggregated by month (Figure 2) and in a sequence index plot (Figure 3). Together these two data displays address our first question, To what extent do households maintain, gain or lose benefits before, during, or after the period of child removal? Figure 2 presents changes in the proportion of households receiving the different benefits over time and Figure 3 displays ordered sequences for the households in each group, allowing greater insight into the transitions from one state to another. For gray-scale display, the three benefit states observed in fewer than 5% of households are collapsed into other categories, leaving five states (1) TANF (only TANF, TANF + GA or TANF + GA + SSI); (2) TANF + SSI; (3) SSI (SSI only or SSI + GA); (4) only GA; or (5) no benefits.[2]

In the most common pattern, the Short Spells of TANF group, between 10% and 40% of households received TANF in a given month. Figure 2 shows that the number of households receiving TANF grows before removal and then descends rapidly. Figure 3 shows short durations of TANF for individual households. Most of the transitions off of TANF were to the "no benefit" state, meaning that these households lost TANF but did not gain other benefits. A small proportion of the households (less than 5%) of the Short Spells of TANF group used GA or SSI after removal.

The Lose TANF group shows a gradual decrease in the monthly TANF receipt rate starting around 9 months prior to the removal (from month − 10 to month − 1) and a very rapid decrease in TANF benefit receipt rate from 70% to 25% quickly after removal (Figure 2). Use of GA increases for this group after removal, but even when including households that gain GA after the removal,

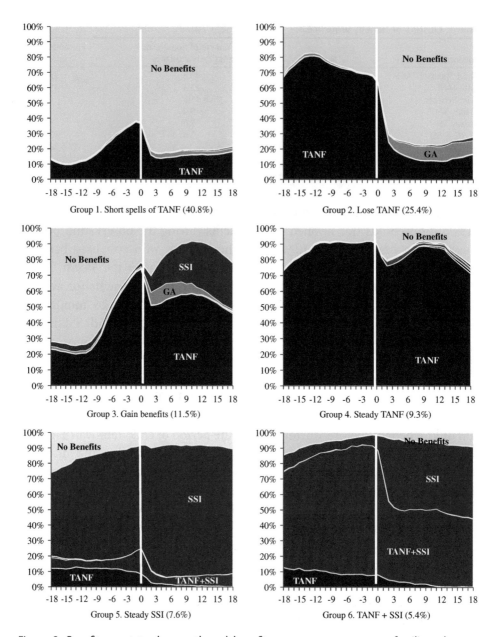

Figure 2. Benefit use states by month and benefit sequence group among families who ever received benefits ($N = 16556$); x-axis indicates month relative to removal and y-axis indicates the percentage of recipient households in group. The removal month (month 0) is indicated with the vertical line.

the benefit usage after removal never recovers to the equivalent level in pre-removal period. By month 18, less than 30% of the Lose TANF group receives any benefit. These overall patterns are echoed in the individual trajectories summarized in Figure 3 for the Lose TANF group. Only a few households in this group are on and off TANF before removal, but few received TANF after the removal. They lose TANF, particularly in the removal month and the

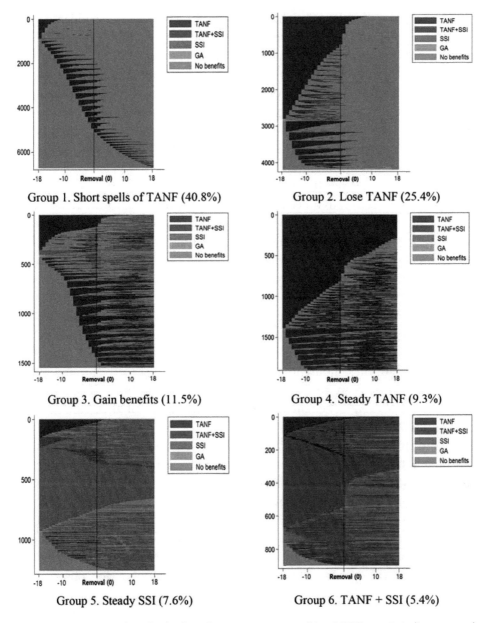

Figure 3. Sequence index plot by benefit sequence group, (N = 16556); x-axis indicates month relative to removal and y-axis indicates the number of recipient households. The removal month (month 0) is indicated with the vertical line.

month after removal. Transitions in Lose TANF group are mostly between TANF and no benefits, but duration of benefit-use sequences are much longer than those in the *Short Spells of TANF*.

The Figure 2 display for the Gain Benefits group shows increasing caseloads over the full observation period and distinctive differences between the pre- and post-removal period. The increase in benefit use before removal is governed by TANF rates, which begin to increase at around 9 months prior to the removal (month − 9). After removal, rates of TANF use drop suddenly then gradually rebuild and fall. GA use increases starting at about 3 months after removal, but then trickles out. The SSI caseload increases in the post-removal months and then levels off with about a third of the Gain Benefits group receiving SSI in the last month of observation. Figure 3 also indicates that TANF is the most common entry point for the Gain Benefits group, with many transitioning onto SSI or GA. These transitions prevailed around the time of the removal. After gaining benefits, most families (80% of this group) maintain receipt through end of the observation window.

Most of the Steady TANF households—about nine out of 10 households in this group—received TANF benefits from 12 months prior to the removal to the removal month (Figure 2). More than half of households in this group received SSI at the beginning of the observation and even more families received SSI after the removal. Even though there was a small drop in TANF receipt right after the removal, it rebounded to be almost equivalent to the pre-removal level within nine months after the removal (month +9). Interruptions of a month or a few months around removal (month 0) for the Steady TANF are common (Figure 3). Only about a fifth of households in Steady TANF have no interruptions of TANF benefit usage throughout the entire 37 months. About a fourth of these households were not on TANF at the beginning of the period, but they began receiving TANF benefits over time. Despite some interruptions of TANF benefit use across time, many of them are able to maintain TANF most of the time observed.

The Steady SSI group generally maintains a high level of SSI participation over time but experienced a temporary decline around the removal (Figure 2). About 10% of *Steady SSI* families received TANF alone or in conjunction with SSI in the months before the removal, but the rate of TANF use dropped to less than 10% by the end of the 37 months (month +18). Figure 3 shows that families in the Steady SSI group tend to continue to receive SSI even after the removal (even if some lost TANF) or moved from TANF to SSI. About half of households in this group receive SSI at the beginning of the observation window (month −18), and about half of those households who had received SSI at the beginning lost SSI benefit at some point around the removal. Many of them, however, regain after or around the removal month. About a third of these households started with no benefits but began to receive SSI over time.

Finally, the display for the TANF + SSI group shows that combining TANF and SSI was more common before removal than after (Figure 2). About 60% of households in this group received both TANF and SSI at the beginning of the 37-month period, a rate that grew to about 80% around the time of removal. Soon after removal, however, concurrent use of both benefits plummeted and use of SSI alone increased, which suggests a loss of TANF benefit. By the end of the period, about half of the TANF + SSI group uses only SSI, and fewer than half receive both benefits. Figure 3 also reflects a pattern of losing TANF benefits for the TANF + SSI group, as many households in this group initially receive both TANF and SSI but by the end most receive only SSI.

Characteristics of benefit sequence groups

Table 2 presents the descriptive characteristics for each cluster membership, addressing our second question about how demographic and case characteristics relate to different benefit sequence groups. This helps to understand the possible association between family characteristics and benefit-use patterns even though it does not establish any causal relation. The last two columns display a summary column of households who *Ever Used Assistance* and who used *No Assistance* in order to compare the differences between families who ever received benefits and families who never received benefits during the 37-month period. *T* tests show that the No Assistance group differs on several dimensions from the *Ever Used Assistance* group and other individual groups who ever received any cash assistance. Households that did not use benefits are older on average with respect to caregivers' and children's ages. They are more likely than other groups to have more child behavior issues and sexual abuse but are less likely to have neglect, physical abuse, and substance abuse. Moreover, they have the highest reunification rate, with a quicker reunification than other groups.

In order to understand which caregiver and case characteristics are associated with different benefit sequence groups, we perform *t* tests comparing clusters against three theoretically motivated reference groups. First, we compare caregivers with Short Spells of TANF, which is the most prevalent group, to those with other patterns. Caregivers who had Short Spells of TANF were younger than those who received SSI (SSI or TANF + SSI) but older than those who lost TANF. Our second reference group is caregivers in the Steady TANF group, which we believe might have been the most prevalent group prior to welfare reform. Caregivers in the Steady TANF group are more likely to have an infant and, on average, have younger children than those in the other TANF groups (Short Spells, Lose TANF, or Gain Benefits). This is not surprising as TANF participants are exempt from work requirements in Washington state—and hence less likely to be sanctioned—for a period after the birth of a child. Both the Short Spells of TANF group and the Steady TANF group were less likely than the Lose TANF group to have neglect as a reason for removal, suggesting that loss of TANF may be associated with increased risk of neglect. Third, we compare caregivers in the No Assistance group, which may be qualitatively different from those who received any benefits. Caregivers and children in the No Assistance group are likely to be older than those in all six benefit sequence groups and the Ever Used group. The No Assistance group is also less likely to have removal reasons caused by primary caregivers but is more likely to have child issue as removal reasons.

Table 2. Demographic and case characteristics by benefit sequence cluster group.

	Short spells of TANF (25.2%)	Lose TANF (15.7%)	Gain Benefits (7.1%)	Steady TANF (5.8%)	Steady SSI (4.7%)	TANF + SSI (3.4%)	Ever used Assistance (61.8%, N = 16,556)	No Assistance (38.2%, N = 10,250)
Caregiver's age	30.9*	29.8*&	30.4*	30.2*	33.0*+&	35.4*+&	30.9*	37.3*+&
Child's age								
Mean	5.8*+	5.7*+	5.9*+	4.8*&	5.8*+	8.4*+&	5.8*	10.9+&
Infant (%)	28.7*+	16.7*+&	17.9*+&	36.4*&	39.1*&	8.5+&	24.8*	9.1+&
1–4 (%)	23.1*+	34.3*+&	33.1*+&	22.8*	14.2*+&	22.7*	26.4*	10.3+&
5–8 (%)	15.5*	20.6*+&	17.8*&	15.1*	11.6&	16.9*	16.8*	9.9+&
9–12 (%)	12.7	14.3	12.7	11.2	11.4	21.5*+&	13.4	14.0
13 and older (%)	20.0*+	14.1*&	18.5*	14.4*&	23.7*+	30.5*+&	18.7*	56.7+&
Race and ethnicity (%)								
White	70.3	68.2*	61.6*+&	70.5	74.4	70.5	69.1*	71.5
African American	7.1*	9.7&	13.1*+&	8.4*	8.4*	12.5*+&	9.0*	5.7*+&
Hispanic	8.2	8.5	11.8*+&	8.5	5.2*+&	4.6*+&	8.3	8.7
Others	12.4*	12.4*	12.4*	11.4	10.7	11.6	12.1*	10.1&
Reasons for removal (%)								
Neglect	55.4*+	65.2*+&	56.0*	59.9*	55.1*	51.7*+	58.2*	29.1+&
Substance Abuse	32.5*	35.1*&	28.1*+&	34.4*	21.5*+&	17.9*+&	31.2*	11.0+&
Physical Abuse	16.6*	14.6*&	15.8	13.5*	13.3*	17.1	15.5*	18.6+&
Sexual Abuse	4.0*	3.7*&	2.7*	2.9*	5.0	5.1	3.8*	6.6+&
Child issue	14.8*+	10.3*&	14.5*	10.8*&	15.0*	20.0*+&	13.5*	45.4+&
Placement outcome (%)								
Reunification	66.3*+	58.3*+&	83.8*+&	71.2*&	50.7*+&	69.1*	65.7*	82.8+&
Within 90 days	42.4*+	32.9*+&	58.0*+&	47.4*&	33.4*+&	49.2*&	41.9*	69.4+&
91–365 days	13.4*	11.5*+	18.4*+&	14.7*	10.1*+&	13.0*	13.4*	8.8+
366 +	10.4*	13.8*+&	7.5*&	9.0*	7.2*&	6.9&	10.4*	4.6+&
Adoption	17.8*+	21.0*+&	7.1*+&	14.4*&	24.9*+&	13.0*&	17.3*	6.1+&
Still in care	12.4*	16.6*+&	6.8*+&	12.2*	18.9*+&	14.5*	13.4*	6.3+&
Aging out	1.4*	2.0*	1.3*	1.2*	2.8&	3.1&	1.7*	3.3*+&
Other	2.1	2.1	1.0&	1.1	2.7+	0.3&	1.8	1.6
Short stay (%)	26.7*	18.8*&	32.3*&	22.8*	21.2*&	29.3*+	24.7*	54.0*+&

Reasons for removal are not exclusive. Short stay indicates whether a child was removed for less than 8 days.
+Significantly different from Steady TANF at p < .05.
&Significantly different from Short Spells of TANF at p < .05.
*Significantly different from No Assistance at p < .05.

Benefit sequence groups and reunification

Our third question is how are benefit sequence groups associated with reunifications outcomes. The bottom panel in Table 2 shows that benefit use is strongly related to reunification patterns. The highest reunification rate, 83.8%, is found among the Gain Benefits group. This group is significantly higher than either the Steady TANF (71.2%) or Short Spells of TANF (66.3%). The Lose TANF group is significantly lower than both reference groups at 58.3%. The Steady SSI group has the lowest overall reunification rate at 50.7%. These correlations between outcomes and TANF use cannot distinguish whether these patterns arise because benefit use is determined in part based on quick or promising reunification, because benefits support family reunification goals, or because of the two combined.

We also examined whether a short removal period is highly associated with the benefit sequence groups we observed. Other child welfare research predicting reunification excludes stays of a week or less because such cases are qualitatively different from longer stays (Hook et al., 2016). We did not exclude short stays because of our focus on dual-system families; high proportions of both short-stay and longer-stay cases use cash assistance. Among families who ever received any cash assistance, 24.7% were short stayers (Table 2). A higher proportion of Gain Benefits cases have short stays relative to those families with Short Spells of TANF and Steady TANF. Lose TANF has lower proportion of short stays (18.8%) than Short Spells of TANF (26.7%). Even though some variations exist among groups for households who used benefits, differences between households who used benefits are small relative to the differences between households who used benefits and the No Assistance group.

Discussion

We examine cash assistance used by families whose children experienced out of home care during the post–welfare reform era. Using administrative data covering the universe of Washington state families who had a child placed out-of-home over the period 1999–2008, we generated distinct groups based on patterns of cash-assistance use. Overall, 61.8% of families who had a child removed from the home received TANF, SSI, or General Assistance either at the point of removal or at some point in the 18 months before or after removal. Six general types of benefit-use patterns characterize these families. Most commonly families had a short spell of TANF (40.8% of those who used any benefit) or lost TANF (25.3%). Other patterns included gaining benefits (11.5%), steady TANF use (9.4%), Steady SSI use (7.6%), and a combination of TANF and SSI (5.4%). In this discussion we note first the limitations of our data and approach, then interpret our findings in light of our original questions and motivation, and finally discuss reasons for both concern and hope stemming from economic and policy events that have happened since our observation period closed.

Study limitations

Findings must be evaluated in light of potential weaknesses in the data and limitations in the scope of the analysis. Data come from only one state, Washington state, which is relatively generous in its benefits and lenient in application of sanctions during the post–welfare reform era (Meyers, Gornick, & Peck, 2001). The state-level administrative data include limited demographic information about the households. Although our focus is on financial supports, the data also do not include information about private support—such as transfers from friends or family—nor locally administered housing subsidies.

Our choice to highlight program participation trajectories of families that experience a child placed out of home deemphasizes other important processes and factors. For instance, our data included only families from whom children were removed; families that come to the attention of the child welfare system but do not experience removal may be less likely to rely on cash assistance or they may be more likely to have stable benefits. Similarly, our analysis does not distinguish between voluntary TANF exits and exits for reasons of sanction or changes in household status. Certainly, exiting TANF because a caregiver is earning money through work is very different from losing benefits and being left without any means of support. However, an analysis of employment and benefit use simultaneously among the same population shows that decreases in benefits are not typically offset by increases in employment for most portions of the caseload (Hook et al., 2016). Because our data are organized around the removal of a focal child, we cannot distinguish between families who maintained benefits because caseworkers applied a concurrent benefit policy or because another child remained in the home. Lastly we examine case outcomes by trajectory group in only a correlational manner, noting which types of removal reasons and outcomes are associated with different patterns of benefit use. This befits the goal of documenting support but does not help untangle the many ways in which case characteristics may result in certain benefit patterns. For instance, based on both policy and our understanding of frontline practice, we believe caseworkers are more likely to request that benefits continue when they judge that the family in question has a good chance of reunification. Future work may investigate the role of policy and frontline workers in different benefit patterns for dual-system families and the causal relationship between different benefit use sequences and renunciation for these families.

Understanding benefit sequences

Limitations notwithstanding, this study offers important new evidence about the limited and tenuous cash assistance used by families in the child welfare system. We believe our findings support two interrelated themes: (a) relatively few families in this post–welfare reform era receive stable cash assistance, but (b) among those who use cash assistance, TANF benefits may promote reunification.

We begin our interpretation of results with the 38.2% of the universe of households with children removed from their caregivers that did not receive cash-assistance benefits during the period surrounding removal. Most of these households (82.8%) reunified, the majority within 90 days. These households may reunify more quickly either because they have greater financial resources or because the primary issue is more often the child's behavioral problems, which is more easily addressed than child neglect.

Among the households who ever received benefits, almost two thirds were characterized as having short spells of TANF (40.8%) or losing TANF (25.3%). This stands in contrast to the small AFDC-era sample in Wells and Guo (2003) in which almost half the families observed received welfare for most or all months prior to removal and about a third of those continued to receive it without interruption for 18 months after removal. We believe our finding reflects a general trend of decreasing and shortened TANF support nationally and within Washington state in the last decade. The number of TANF parent-headed households (i.e., excluding child-only cases) for caseloads in Washington state fell over our observation period, from 68,707 in January 1998 to 40,894 in December 2009, an overall decrease of just over 40% (Author calculations based on U.S. Department of Health & Human Services, n.d.). Nationally the drop was more dramatic, down almost 60% over the same time period. These trends reflect the policy goals of the 1996 welfare reform—to make aid "temporary"—and are consistent with short spells of TANF use observed among the general population of recipients (Cancian, Meyer, & Wu, 2005). This suggests that TANF receipt would have likely dropped for any cross-section of poor families observed for 3 years over our time frame.

National tightening of TANF does not, however, account for the sharp decreases in TANF use observed in the months immediately following child removal. Rather we believe this reflects interactions with systems causing parents to lose TANF. Across all six types of benefit use, a drop in TANF cash use is evident following removal. This drop is most dramatic in the Lose TANF group. Households who lose TANF are also less likely to reunify relative to almost all of the other groups. This finding is consistent with prior studies showing correlations between welfare loss and worse child welfare outcomes, including greater risk of child welfare involvement (Shook, 1999) and lower reunification after removal (Wells & Guo, 2006); the only group with lower reunification rates than the Lose TANF group is the Steady SSI group, 7.6% of benefit recipient. We believe that severe caregiver disabilities explain the low reunification rate for the SSI group). The most prevalent group, Short Spells of TANF, reunified at a lower rate than households who did not use benefits or those categorized as Gain Benefits or Steady TANF. This is consistent with

AFDC-era work by Barbara Needell and colleagues (Needell, Cuccaro-Alamin, Brookhart, & Lee, 1999), which found that families with interruptions in benefit use were at greater risk of continued abuse and neglect.

Of course, two different causal stories can explain the co-occurrence of low rates of reunification and a loss of TANF benefits within a group. Losing benefits may further destabilize caregivers, making it harder for them to meet requirements for reunification. For instance, losing benefits may mean a caregiver loses housing or is unable to afford transportation to required appointments. On the other hand, these may be cases with more severe issues, in which caseworker assessments suggest that reunification is unlikely and, hence, removing the caregiver from the TANF rolls is warranted. We believe both patterns likely occurred, but the low rates of TANF use after removal suggest that many households in this group may have experienced material hardship while working toward and after reunification. Although the Lose TANF group had the second-lowest reunification rate, over half of this group (58.3%) did reunify, a third within 90 days of removal. These might have been households who successfully gained employment or found private assistance such as support from relatives. However, while over 70% of Lose TANF households received cash assistance prior to removal, only a minority (less than a third) did so after removal.

In contrast to those who lost benefits, the highest rate of reunification was observed for households who gained benefits over the observation window. The Gain Benefits group's reunification rate (83.8%) was statistically equivalent to the relatively wealthier No Assistance group. We believe this group illustrates potential pathways whereby the convergence of cash assistance and child welfare supports families. Many of these households started TANF in the 6 months prior to removal or gained SSI benefits after removal. These may be cases in which the first point of child welfare contact was several months before removal. In such situations, caseworkers may have coordinated services, including TANF, to stabilize and support families. Alternatively, families may have come to the attention of the child welfare system because they applied for TANF and were hence more visible to the system (Shook Slack et al., 2003), but the high reunification rate suggests that intervention may have been relatively brief and helpful.

Steady TANF use, the benefit group that characterizes 9.4% of the benefit recipients, also has a high reunification rate of 71.2%. We believe these are largely young families. Over a third of focal children in the Steady TANF families were infants and the average child age for this group was the lowest across all groups. Child age also explains why these families were able to maintain TANF benefits, as Washington state exempted parents from TANF work requirements for participants caring for a child under four months old for cumulative 12 months in a recipients' life time during the study period.

In sum, we believe our findings support some of the concerns about how well dual-system families would fare post–welfare reform (McGowan & Walsh,

2000; Ward Doran & Roberts, 2002). The higher-than-average reunification rates among households who received steady TANF or got connected to benefits (Gain Benefits) suggests that benefits were related to—and we believe assisted in—reunification. Relative to these groups, the patterns of benefit receipt made most common by welfare reform, short TANF spells or losing benefits, were associated with lower rates of reunification.

Recent changes and future directions

Our study period ended during the waxing months of the Great Recession. Recession-driven changes to state budgets suggest that the transience of cash assistance has become even more problematic for parents in need of support. However, recent changes to TANF policies in Washington state have also extended more stable support to dual-system families.

Despite a temporary federally funded increase, TANF support has become less generous and more tenuous since the period observed in our study. Rising unemployment during the Great Recession increased need for cash assistance just as falling tax rolls limited states' abilities to respond. A TANF emergency fund in the American Reinvestment and Recovery Act of 2009 provided 2 years of extra support for state spending on core TANF functions including basic cash assistance and subsidized employment (U.S. Administration for Children and Families, 2012). This temporarily buffeted state budgets and allowed state administrations to partially respond to increased need. In Washington state, the TANF caseload increased 30% over the period 2008–2011 (Patton, Ford Shah, Felver, & Beall, 2015). However, the federal emergency fund ended in 2010, with TANF rolls again dropping sharply nationwide, despite lingering high employment (Hall, 2015). A national scan of state administrators suggests that many states restricted TANF benefits or cut staffing after 2010 (Brown & Derr, 2015). Washington state reduced the TANF payment standards and tightened time limits in 2011. By 2014, Washington state spending on TANF benefits had dropped by 32% relative to 2008, the last pre-Recession year (author calculations using Pavetti, 2015). State caseloads, which had grown to 65,140 households after Recession, dropped to 42,549 households, well below the pre-Recession level of 55,610 (Patton et al, 2015).

Although federal funds temporarily protected TANF, state GA had no such backstop. In the Great Recession and its immediate aftermath, over a third of the 30 states that still offered some type of general assistance as of 2011 had recently cut back or were considering restrictive measures (Schott & Cho, 2011). Washington state numbered among those that cut GA. In 2011—2 years after the end of our observation period—the state replaced GA with a more restricted program with stricter time limits and a greater emphasis on disability. This subsequent program was further limited a year later and renamed Aged, Blind or Disabled (ABD). The 2009 GA caseload served an average of 34,992 persons per month with an average benefit of $308. In 2013, ABD served 38% fewer persons

(22,840) with an average transfer of $172. Given that our study concludes before the retrenchment of GA in 2011, we expect that dual-system families now are more likely to have more economic hardships than before because some cases in TANF benefit loss are not replaced with GA participation.

Policy and agency changes in how systems serve low-income, dual-system families may help counteract these larger trends. Although TANF is typically predicated on having a child in the home, program options allow state discretion in whether caregivers from whom children are removed can continue to receive TANF benefits if reunification is expected to take place. Temporary absence policy in Washington state allows benefits to continue if reunification is anticipated within 180 days, and benefits are provided concurrently if the child moves to another household receiving a TANF grant. Washington state put these policies in place in August 2008, after the latest removals in our data. At the same time, HSD took a "significant step forward in the active collaboration between" the HSD subagencies of Economic Services, which implements TANF, and Children's Administration, responsible for child welfare (Dori Shoji, HSD, written communication, November 3, 2014). The two administrations share case management system information with each other's caseworkers and supervisors, although not all staff members have received training. Given this study's evidence of a sharp drop-off of TANF use within 3 months of removal, these efforts seem to have the potential to stabilize families. Indeed, an analysis of concurrent benefit recipients with a comparison group by observable characteristics showed that those caregivers who continued to receive TANF benefits after removal reunified faster and at a higher rate (Marshall, Beall, Mancuso, Yette, & Felver, 2013).

In sum, this analysis documents that support from public assistance programs is important to families involved with the child welfare system. Policies that stabilize support during the tumultuous time surrounding a child's removal from the home and casework practices that help connect families to benefits for which they might be eligible can promote reunification. State policy makers should consider these conclusions in light of how their systems serve dual-system families.

Notes

1. Youth ages 12 to 18 who spend a short period in residential treatment constitute most of the second group; these placements are often voluntary in that parents seek help (Marcenko et al., 2012). We believe it is appropriate to include these cases in the analysis as they are also likely to be poor or at risk of poverty (wealthier households are more likely to draw on private resources to treat youths' behavioral needs).
2. Color plots with all eight benefit combination states are available in Appendix 1.

Acknowledgments

The U.S. Department of Health and Human Services/Administration for Children and Families funded data acquisition through a grant to the University of Washington West Coast Poverty

Center and final writing through Romich's Family Self Sufficiency and Stability Research Scholars award (90PD0279). Partial support for this research came from a Eunice Kennedy Shriver National Institute of Child Health and Human Development research infrastructure grant to the Center for Studies in Demography & Ecology at the University of Washington (R24 HD042828). The authors wish to acknowledge the contributions of Partners for Our Children, the Washington State Department of Social and Health Services (DSHS) Research and Data Analysis Division, DSHS's Children's Administration, and DSHS's Economic Services Administration. We thank Mark Eddy, Susan Barkan, Dori Shoji, and David Stillman for their assistance and thoughtful comments on this manuscript.

References

Abbott, A., & Hrycak, A. (1990). Measuring resemblance in sequence data?: An optimal matching analysis of musicians' careers. *American Journal of Sociology*, *96*(1), 144–185.

Aisenbrey, S., & Fasang, A. E. (2010). New life for old ideas: The "second wave" of sequence analysis bringing the "course" back into the life course. *Sociological Methods and Research*, *38*(3), 420–462.

Berrick, J. D. (1999). Entitle to what? Welfare and child welfare in a shifting policy environment. *Children and Youth Service Review*, *21*(9/10), 709–717.

Brown, E., & Derr, M. K. (2015). Serving Temporary Assistance for Needy Families (TANF) recipients in a post-recession environment (#2015–05). Washington, DC: U.S. Department of Health and Human Services, Administration for Children and Families, Office of Planning, Research and Evaluation.

Brzinsky-Fay, C. (2007). Lost in transition? Labour market entry sequences of school leavers in Europe. *European Sociological Review*, *23*(4), 409–422.

Brzinsky-Fay, C., Kohler, U., & Luniak, M. (2006). Sequence analysis with Stata. *Stata Journal*, *6*(4), 435–460.

Cancian, M., Meyer, D., & Wu, C. (2005). After the revolution: Welfare patterns since TANF implementation. *Social Work Research*, *29*(4), 199–214.

Committee on Ways and Means, U.S. House of Representatives. (1996). Summary of welfare reforms made by Public Law 104-193 the Personal Responsibility and Work Opportunity Reconciliation Act and associated legislation. U.W. Government Printing Office.

Connell-Carrick, K. (2003). A critical review of the empirical literature: Identifying risk factors for child neglect. *Child and Adolescent Social Work*, *20*(5), 389–425.

Courtney, M. E., Dworsky, A., Piliavin, I., & Zinn, A. (2005). Involvement of TANF applicant families with Child Welfare Services. *Social Service Review*, *79*(1), 119–157.

Ehrle, J., Scarcella, C. A., & Geen, R. (2004). Teaming up: Collaboration between welfare and child welfare agencies since welfare reform. *Children and Youth Services Review*, *26*(3), 265–285.

Frame, L. (1999). Suitable Homes Revisited: An historical look at child protection and welfare reform. *Children and Youth Services Review, 21*(9/10), 719–754.

Gabadinho, A., Ritschard, G., Studer, M., & Nicolas, S. M. (2010). *Mining sequence data in R with the TraMineR package.* Geneva, Switzerland: University of Geneva. Retrieved from http://mephisto.unige.ch/pub/TraMineR/doc/1.4/TraMineR-1.4-Users-Guide.pdf

Geen, R., Fender, L., Leos-Urbel, J., Markowitz, T., & the Urban Institute (2001). *Welfare reform's effect on child welfare caseloads.* Washington, DC: Urban Institute.

Halpin, B., & Chan, T. W. (1998). Careers as sequences?: An optimal matching analysis of work-life histories. *European Journal of Sociological Review, 14*(2), 111–130.

Hall, R. (2015). *TANF in the great recession: Weakness in the safety net* (TANF 101). Washington, DC: Center for Law and Social Policy.

Havlicek, J. (2010). Patterns of movement in foster care: An optimal matching analysis. *Social Service Review, 84*(3), 403–435.

Hook, J. L., Romich, J. L., Lee, J. S., Marcenko, M. O., Kang, J. Y. (2016). Trajectories of economic disconnection among families in the child welfare system. *Social Problems, 63*(2/May), 161–179.

Kortenkamp, K., Geen, R., & Stagner, M. (2004). The role of welfare and work in predicting foster care reunification rates for children of welfare recipients. *Children and Youth Services Review, 26,* 577–590.

Marcenko, M. O., Hook, J. L., Romich, J. L., & Lee, J. (2012). Multiple jeopardy: Poor, economically disconnected, and child welfare involved. *Child Maltreatment, 17*(3), 195–206.

Marshall, D. B., Beall, K., Mancuso, D., Yette, R., & Felver, B. (2013). Effect of TANF concurrent benefits on the reunification of children following placement in out-of-home care (RDA report 11.198). Olympia, WA: Washington State Department of Social and Health Services Research and Data Analysis Division.

McGowan, B. G., & Walsh, E. M. (2000). Policy challenges for child welfare in the new century. *Child Welfare, 79*(1), 11–27.

Meyers, M. K., Gornick, J. C., & Peck, L. (2001). Packaging support for low income families. *Journal of Policy Analysis and Management, 20*(3), 457–486.

Needell, B., Cuccaro-Alamin, S., Brookhart, A., & Lee, S. (1999). Transitions from AFDC to child welfare in California. *Children and Youth Service Review, 21*(9/10), 815–841.

Patton, D., Ford Shah, M., Felver, B. E. M., & Beall, K. (2015). TANF caseload decline (Report to the Washington state [HSD] Economic Services Administration). Office of the Assistant Secretary and the Community Services Division. Olympia, WA: Author.

Pavetti, L. (2015). TANF spending spreadsheet (2014 data). Washington, DC: Center for Budget and Policy Priorities. Retrieved from http://www.cbpp.org/research/family-income-support/how-states-use-federal-and-state-funds-under-the-tanf-block-grant

Paxson, C., & Waldfogel, J. (2002). Work, welfare, and child maltreatment. *Journal of Labor Economics, 20*(3), 435–474.

Pelton, L. H. (1989). *For reasons of poverty.* New York, NY: Praeger.

Pecora, P. J., Whittaker, J. K., Maluccio, A. N., Barth, R. P., & Plotnick, R. D. (2009). *The child welfare challenge: Policy, practice, and research.* New Brunswick, Canada: Aldine Transaction.

Piccarreta, R., & Lior, O. (2010). Exploring sequences?: A graphical tool based on multi-dimensional scaling. *Journal of Royal Statstical Society, 173*(1), 165–184.

Pollock, G. (2014). Holistic trajectories?: A study of combined employment, housing and family careers by multiple-sequence analysis. *Journal of the Royal Statistical Society, 170*(1), 167–183.

Rivausx, S. L., James, K., Wittenstron, K., Baumann, D., Sheets, J., Henry, J., & Jeffries, V. (2008). The Intersection of Race, Poverty, and Risk: Understanding the decision to provide services to clients and to remove children. *Child Welfare, 87*(2), 151–168.

Schmidt, L., & Sevak, P. (2004). AFDC, SSI, and welfare reform aggressiveness: Caseload reductions versus caseload shifting. *Journal of Human Resources, 39*(3), 792–812.

Schott, L., & Cho, C. (2011). *General assistance programs: Safety net weakening despite increased need.* Washington, DC: Center on Budget and Policy Priorities. Retrieved from http://www.

cbpp.org/research/family-income-support/general-assistance-programs-safety-net-weakeni
ng-despite-increased

Schott, L., & Hill, M. (2015). *State general assistance programs are weakening despite increased need.* Washington, DC: Center on Budget and Policy Priorities. Retrieved from http://www. cbpp.org/research/family-income-support/state-general-assistance-programs-are-weakening-despite-increased

Simonson, J., Gordo, L. R., & Titova, N. (2011). Changing employment patterns of women in Germany: How do baby boomers differ from older cohorts? A comparison using sequence analysis. *Advances in Life Course Research, 16*(2), 65–82.

Slack, K. S. (1999). Does the loss of welfare income increase the risk of involvement with the child welfare system? *Children and Youth Services Review, 21*(9/10), 781–814.

Slack, K. S., Holl, J. L., Lee, B. J., McDaniel, M., Altenbernd, L., & Stevens, A. B. (2003). Child protective intervention in the context of welfare reform. *Journal of Policy Analysis and Management, 22*(4), 517–536.

Slack, K. S., Lee, B. J., & Berger, L. M. (2007). Do welfare sanctions increase child protection system involvement? A cautious answer. *Social Service Review, 81*(2), 207–228.

U.S. Administration for Children and Families. (2012). Background information about the TANF Emergency Fund. Retrieved from http://www.acf.hhs.gov/programs/ofa/resource/background-information-about-the-tanf-emergency-fund

U.S. Committee on Ways and Means, U.S. House of Representatives. (1996). Summary of welfare reforms made by Public Law 104-193 the Personal Responsibility and Work Opportunity Reconciliation Act and associated legislation (WMCP: 104-15). Washington, DC; U.S. Government Printing Office.

U.S. Social Security Administration, Office of Retirement and Disability Policy. (2014). Monthly statistical snapshot, May 2014. Retreived from http://www.ssa.gov/policy/docs/quickfacts/s tat_snapshot/2014-05.html

U.S. Department of Health and Human Services, Office of Assistant Secretary for Planning and Evaluation. (2000). *Dynamics of Children's Movement Among the AFDC, Medicaid, and Foster Care Programs Prior to Welfare Reform: 1995–1996.* Washington, DC. Retrieved from https://aspe.hhs.gov/execsum/dynamics-childrens-movement-among-afdc-medicaid-and-foster-care-programs-prior-welfare-reform-1995–1996

Waldfogel, J. (2004). Welfare reform and the child welfare system. *Children and Youth Services Review, 26*(10), 919–939.

Wamhoff, S., & Wiseman, M. (2006). The TANF/SSI connection. *Social Security Bulletin, 66*(4), 21–36.

Ward Doran, M. B., & Roberts, D. E. (2002). Welfare reform and families in the child welfare system. *Maryland Law Review, 61*(2), 386–436.

Wells, K., & Guo, S. (2003). Mothers's welfare and work income and reunification with children in foster care. *Children and Youth Services Review, 25*(3), 203–224.

Wells, K., & Guo, S. (2004). Reunification of foster children before and after welfare reform. *Social Service Review, 78*(1), 74–95.

Wells, K., & Guo, S. (2006). Welfare reform and child welfare outcomes: A multiple-cohort study. *Children and Youth Services Review, 28*(8), 941–960.

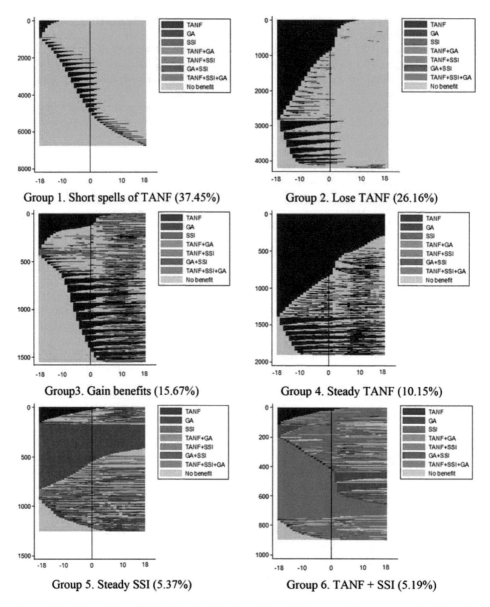

Appendix 1. Colored Benefit Use States by Month and Benefit Sequence Group among Families who ever received benefits ($N = 16556$); x-axis indicates month relative to removal and y-axis indicates the number of recipient households. The removal month (month 0) is indicated with the vertical line.

Antipsychotic Use and Foster Care Placement Stability Among Youth With Attention-Deficit Hyperactivity/Disruptive Behavior Disorders

Ming-Hui Tai, Terry V. Shaw, and Susan dosReis

ABSTRACT

The objective of this study was to investigate the association between antipsychotic initiation and placement transitions among youth in foster care with attention-deficit/hyperactivity disorder and other disruptive behavior disorders (ADHD/DBD). Data were obtained from child welfare administrative records and Medicaid claims in one Mid-Atlantic state from January 1, 2010, through March 31, 2014. Cox proportional hazard model was conducted to estimate the risk of time to first placement transition during the 180-day follow-up among new antipsychotic users and propensity score matched nonusers. Results showed youth initiating antipsychotics had no significant reduction in foster placement transitions within the 180-day follow up (Hazard Ratio = 1.1; 95% CI = 0.7–1.6). Although antipsychotics are widely used for aggressive behaviors, a better understanding of clinical management of youth in foster care is needed to promote stable foster placement.

The more than 400,000 youth in the United States in foster care represent a vulnerable population with higher mental healthcare costs and greater service needs relative to other youth in the community (Johnson, Silver, & Wulczyn, 2013; Rubin, O'Reilly, Luan, & Localio, 2007; U.S. Department of Health and Human Services, Administration for Children and Families, Administration on Children, Youth and Families, Children's Bureau, 2014). Nearly half of youth who are placed in foster care have significant behavioral problems (Newton, Litrownik, & Landsverk, 2000), such as attention-deficit/hyperactivity disorder (ADHD), conduct disorder, impulse control disorder, and oppositional defiant disorder. Moreover, behavioral problems are a key reason for foster care placement disruptions (Barber, Delfabbro, & Cooper, 2001; Fisher, Stoolmiller, Mannering, Takahashi, & Chamberlain, 2011), and it is well-documented that multiple placement transitions could lead to negative outcomes such as poor academic attainment, lack of social engagement, and continued mental health problems in adulthood (Barber et al., 2001; Carnochan, Moore, & Austin, 2013;

Color versions of one or more of the figures in the article can be found online at www.tandfonline.com/wpcw.

Jonson-Reid & Barth, 2000; Leathers, 2006; Taber & Proch, 1987; University of California Davis Extension, The Center for Human Services, 2008).

Management of behavioral disorders is clinically challenging, and psychotropic medications commonly are prescribed to manage aggressive and irritable behaviors (Cooper, Hickson, Fuchs, Arbogast, & Ray, 2004; Crystal, Olfson, Huang, Pincus, & Gerhard, 2009a; Loy, Merry, Hetrick, & Stasiak, 2012; Olfson, Blanco, Liu, Wang, & Correll, 2012; Rubin, Feudtner, Localio, & Mandell, 2009). Moreover, rates of antipsychotic use are also disproportionately higher for youth in foster care relative to other Medicaid-insured or privately insured youth (dosReis et al., 2011; Olfson, Blanco, Liu, Moreno, & Laje, 2006; Rubin et al., 2007; Zito, Burcu, Ibe, Safer, & Magder, 2013). Treatment Recommendations for the Use of Antipsychotics for Aggressive Youth (TRAAY) published by the American Academy of Child and Adolescent Psychiatry (AACAP) state that antipsychotics could follow an initial trial with stimulants for youth with aggression or severe ADHD (Pappadopulos et al., 2003). However, studies from national survey data have reported that antipsychotic use among this vulnerable population has increased at a rate greater than other psychotropic drugs, suggesting more youth are initiating treatment with an antipsychotic (Cooper et al., 2006; John M. Eisenberg Center for Clinical Decisions and Communications Science, 2007) rather than through the recommended process of an initial trial with a stimulant. For example, one state Medicaid data has showed new antipsychotic users nearly doubled from 0.23% in 1996 to 0.45% in 2001 (Cooper et al., 2004). Other research has found the prevalence of antipsychotic use among youth in foster care nationally increased from 8.9% in 2002 to 11.8% in 2007, which exceeded the 5.2% to 5.9% increase in psychotropic use during the same time (Rubin et al., 2009).

Antipsychotics are prescribed more commonly for ADHD, conduct disorders, and depression/anxiety, than for schizophrenia, bipolar disorder, autism, and Tourette's disorder (Crystal, Olfson, Huang, Pincus, & Gerhard, 2009b). Prior research studied the use of antipsychotics among Medicaid-enrolled youth in a Mid-Atlantic state across a decade. The study found the increase in antipsychotic users was greatest among youth with ADHD (7.3% to 20.2%) and with other disruptive behavior disorders (9.6% in 1997 to 22.1% in 2006) (Zito et al., 2013). The use of antipsychotics for disruptive behavioral disorders among youth is concerning because antipsychotic treatment for pediatric populations has limited U.S. Food and Drug Administration (FDA) approved indications. Approved indications include schizophrenia, autism, Tourette's disorder, and bipolar disorder, and the rise in use of antipsychotics has occurred disproportionally for non-FDA approved conditions (Olfson et al., 2006; 2012; Rubin et al., 2009; Zito et al., 2013).

Despite the growing use of antipsychotics to manage youth behaviors, no study has investigated the association between antipsychotic initiation and placement stability among youth in foster care. Theory and practice would suggest that if behavioral problems increase the risk of foster placement transitions also increases. If antipsychotics are effective in managing aggressive behaviors, then antipsychotic medication could have an influence on placement transition via management of problematic behaviors that lead to frequent transitions. The objective of this study is to examine the association between antipsychotic initiation and foster care placement transitions among youth with ADHD and other disruptive behavior disorders (ADHD/DBD). It was hypothesized that youth who initiated antipsychotic medication would be less likely to experience a placement transition and the time to a placement transition would be longer compared with youth who did not receive antipsychotics. The study was reviewed and approved by the Institutional Review Board for the academic institution and each respective state agency. The study used de-identified data that did not include social security number, Medicaid identification number, or any other personal identifier.

Patients and methods

Data source

Child welfare administrative records and Medicaid claims for mental health services in one Mid-Atlantic state were obtained through ongoing evaluation contracts to examine the association between antipsychotic initiation and placement stability among youth in foster care. Data privacy agreements prohibit the disclosure of the geographic location. All records of youth in out-of-home placement at any time from January 1, 2010, through March 31, 2014, in one Mid-Atlantic state were identified and then linked to Medicaid claims to characterize any mental health treatment provided during the youth's time in foster care. The use of different administrative data systems is necessary as neither system alone contains the sufficient information to investigate the association between antipsychotic initiation and child welfare outcomes, such as placement stability.

Child welfare administrative records provided information on youth demographics and child welfare system involvement, including the youth's age, gender, race, the date of removal from and date of return to the home of origin, and the reasons for removal (i.e., abuse, neglect). Foster care information included the placement entry and exit dates, placement type (i.e., family home/kinship, group home, foster home, and institution), and spell number (i.e., the number of times a youth had been removed from the home).

The foster placement file was merged with two separate Medicaid claims files: pharmacy and mental health claims. Pharmacy claims for all prescriptions dispensed in outpatient pharmacies were used to identify youth who received psychotropic medications anytime during 2010–2013. Psychotropic medications, classified by therapeutic class, included antipsychotics (first-generation:

chlorpromazine, fluphenazine, haloperidol, loxapine, and perphenazine; second-generation: aripiprazole, asenapine, clozapine, iloperidone, olanzapine, paliper-idone, quetiapine, risperidone, and ziprasidone), ADHD medications (stimulants and atomoxetine), antidepressants, and mood stabilizers (lithium and anticonvulsants: carbamazepine, valproic acid, gabapentin, lamotrigine, and oxcarbazepine).

Public mental health claims for inpatient, emergency department, and outpatient services claims were used to identify mental health-related visits; defined as a claim associated with an *International Classification of Diseases, Ninth Revision* (ICD-9) diagnostic code for a psychiatric disorder. The ICD-9 codes were classified into the following groups: schizophrenia (295), bipolar disorder (296.00–296.10; 296.4–296.8), depression (296.20–296.35), autism (299), anxiety disorder (300.00–300.29 and 301.4), Tourette's syndrome (307.2), conduct disorder (312.00–313.89), impulsive control (312.3), oppositional defiant disorder (313.8), ADHD (314), and mental retardation (317–319). Psychotherapy was identified from mental health claims using Current Procedural Terminology (CPT) code. It defined as any individual, family, or group psychotherapy in the 180 days prior to the index date.

Study population

A new user design was implemented to identify a cohort of youth in foster care who initiated antipsychotic treatment during the study period. A new antipsychotic user cohort was identified from the population of youth age 21 years or younger who were in foster care and who received an antipsychotic prescription (i.e., index date) during calendar years 2010–2013. Inclusion criteria were: (a) 180 days of continuous foster care enrollment preceding the index date, (b) 210 days of continuous foster care enrollment following the index date, and (c) no antipsychotic medication 180 days prior to the index date. In order to focus on antipsychotic use for disruptive behavior disorders, exclusions were made if a youth had a diagnosis of schizophrenia and bipolar disorder. The cohort selection is illustrated in Figure 1.

Potential controls for the comparison cohort (i.e., nonuser) were selected among youth who did not receive antipsychotic prescription at any time during calendar years 2010–2013. However, nonusers may or may not have received psychotropic medications other than antipsychotics. To assign an index date to each nonuser, a new user was randomly selected and his/her index date was assigned to a nonuser. This approach avoids imbalance of the time distribution between new users and nonusers and reduces potential selection bias (Zhou, Rahme, Abrahamowicz, & Pilote, 2005). Once an index date was assigned, the same inclusion criteria were also applied to the nonusers: (a) 180 days of continuous foster care enrollment preceding the index date, and (b) 210 days of continuous foster care enrollment following the index date.

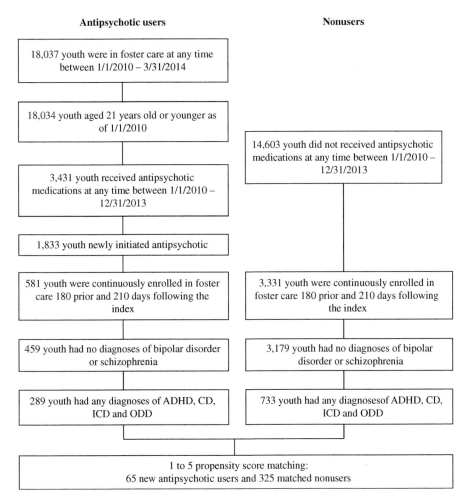

Figure 1. Cohort selection for new antipsychotic users and nonusers among youth in foster care. ADHD = attention-deficit/hyperactivity disorder; ODD = oppositional defiant disorder; CD = conduct disorder; ICD = impulse control disorder.

Covariates

Demographic, clinical, and foster placement characteristics served as covariates. Demographic characteristics included age as of January 2010, gender, and race (white, black/African American, and others). Psychiatric diagnoses identified from mental health claims, assessed in the 180 days preceding the index date, were categorized as any internalizing disorders (anxiety, depression, and post-traumatic stress disorder [PTSD]), mood disorders, and developmental disorders (autism, mental retardation, and other pervasive developmental disorders). The psychiatric diagnostic categories were not mutually exclusive. Foster care placement characteristics, including number of lifetime spells, reasons for foster placement (i.e., abuse, neglect), number of placement transitions, placement type, and the age at first removal from his/her biological family, were assessed 180 days preceding the index date.

Primary outcome

The primary outcomes were foster placement transition, coded as a binary indicator of any transition, and time to first placement transition, both assessed from day 31 to 210 following the index date. A 30-day lag between the index date and start of follow-up was implemented to reinforce the temporality between antipsychotics and placement transitions as well as to avoid confounding from administrative transition processes that may have been occurring at the time of the antipsychotic initiation.

Statistical analysis

To balance characteristics between new users and nonusers, propensity score (PS) matching was implemented using greedy matching algorithms (Parsons, 2004). The conditional probability of being new users was calculated given the covariates, which are either related to antipsychotic initiation and placement transition or placement transition only. The stepwise variable selection algorithm was used to develop a good predictive model of antipsychotic initiation. With c-statistic of 0.862, variables in the final PS model included age, clinical profile 180-days prior to the index date (any externalizing disorder, internalizing disorder, ADHD medication use, antidepressant use, mood stabilizer use, and number of hospitalizations), and foster care characteristics such as any physical/sexual abuse, age of removal from his/her biological family, and foster care placement type in the 180-days prior to the index date. The final cohort included 5 nonusers for every 1 new antipsychotic user. The baseline characteristics are presented in Table 1. The new antipsychotic users and nonusers were compared initially using chi-square tests for categorical data and t tests for continuous data. A time-to-event model was used to follow subjects from the day 31 following the index date to first placement transition or the end of the study period, whichever occurred first.

The relationship between antipsychotic initiation and placement transition is subject to reverse causality. To address the potential confounder that multiple placement transitions may underlie the reason for antipsychotic initiation, the cohort was restricted to youth who had no more than two placement transitions in the 180 days preceding the index date. Cox proportional hazard models were used to estimate hazard ratios (HRs) associated with antipsychotic initiation. The Cox proportional hazards assumption was confirmed visually by graphing the log $(-\log[\text{survival}])$ against $\log(t)$ curves and statistically by testing the interaction terms between log time and antipsychotic initiation.

Sensitivity analysis

We used a 6-month window to identify new users, but in fact a youth may have received an antipsychotic prior to the 6-month window. Thus, misclassification

Table 1. Comparison of characteristics among new antipsychotic users and nonusers in the study cohort.

	New User N = 65		Nonusers N = 325		Overall N = 390	
	N	%	N	%	N	%
Demographic characteristics						
Age (mean, SD)	14.6 (4.0)		14.6 (3.9)		14.6 (3.9)	
Age (yrs)						
≤5	2	3.1	11	3.4	13	3.3
6–10	8	12.3	40	12.3	48	12.3
11–15	23	35.4	106	32.6	129	33.1
16–21	32	49.2	168	51.7	200	51.3
Gender						
Male	33	50.8	195	60.0	228	58.5
Female	32	49.2	130	40.0	162	41.5
Race						
White	15	23.1	54	16.6	69	17.7
Black/African American	48	73.8	264	81.2	312	80.0
Others	2	3.1	7	2.2	9	2.3
*Clinical Characteristics**						
Psychiatric diagnosis						
Externalizing disorders	65	100.0	325	100.0	390	100.0
Internalizing disorders	26	40.0	119	36.6	145	37.2
Developmental disorders	2	3.1	13	4.0	15	3.8
Psychotherapy	9	13.8	29	8.9	38	9.7
Service utilization						
Any hospitalization[†]	10	15.4	35	10.8	45	11.5
Any emergency department visit	4	6.2	11	3.4	15	3.8
*Foster Care Characteristics**						
Age when the child was removed from home (mean, SD)						
	8.8 (4.9)		8.8 (4.7)		8.8 (4.7)	
Reasons for entry foster care						
Physical/Sexual abuse	18	27.7	89	27.4	107	27.4
Number of spells (mean, SD)	1.3 (0.6)		1.4 (0.7)		1.4 (0.7)	
Any foster placement transition[†]	23	13.7	105	32.3	128	32.8
Type of placement among child with any transition						
Family home and kinship	5	7.7	25	7.7	30	7.7
Group home and Institution	8	12.3	33	10.2	41	10.5
Foster home	14	21.5	57	17.5	71	18.2

*Characteristics were from 180-day prior to the index date; [†]$p < .05$.

could occur when a youth is actually a prevalent user not a new user. Thus, the sensitivity analysis was conducted to test whether the study results were robust given the possibility of misclassifying new antipsychotic users. A 270-day look-back period of no antipsychotic use prior to the index date was used. Statistical significance was determined by two-sided p-values at the 5% significance level. All analyses were conducted using SAS 9.3 (SAS Institute Inc., Cary, NC).

Results

Of the 18,034 youth age 21 years and younger and enrolled in foster care at any time during the study period, 3,431 (19.0%) received at least one antipsychotic prescription, of which 1,833 (53.4%) were new antipsychotic users. Of the 581 new users who were continuously in foster care 180 days before and 210 days after the index date, 289 had a diagnosis of ADHD/DBD in the absence of schizophrenia or bipolar disorder. The incidence of antipsychotic use among foster youth with ADHD/DBD and no psychosis-related disorders was 16 per 1,000 (i.e., 289 new users out of 18,034 youth in foster care during the study period). Approximately 35% of the new antipsychotic users had any prior use of other psychotropic medications 180 days before initiating antipsychotics. Of these new antipsychotic users, risperidone (46.8%), aripiprazole (24.3%), and quetiapine (21.9%) were commonly prescribed. Moreover, 48% of these new users received ADHD medications and 44% received antidepressants in the 180 days prior to the index date (data not shown).

Characteristics of the matched sample

Table 1 displays the sample characteristics of new users ($n = 65$) and propensity score matched nonusers ($n = 325$). Overall, the youth sample ($n = 390$) was on average 15 (± 3.9) years-old, 58.5% male, and 80.0% black/African American. Just more than one-third (37.2%) had an internalizing disorder, 11.5% had any hospitalization, and 3.8% had an emergency department visit 180 days prior to the index date. The mean age at removal from his/her biological family was 9 (± 4.7) years old, 27.4% had any physical/sexual abuse, and 32.8% had at least one placement transition in the 180 days prior to the index date.

Time to placement transition

Table 2 illustrates the percentage of youth who experienced placement transitions and mean time to first transition between new antipsychotic users and nonusers. During the follow up period, an approximately equal proportion of new users and nonusers experienced at least one placement transition during the study follow-up. Among youth who had a placement transition, the mean time to the first transition was 109 $\pm$ 48 days for new users and 113 $\pm$ 54 days for nonusers. There was no statistically significant difference between the groups with regard to placement transition or mean time to first transition during the180-day follow up between days 31 and 210 after the index prescription.

The Kaplan-Meier curves for time to first transition for new users and nonusers are displayed in Figure 2. In the first two months of follow-up, the

Table 2. Assessment of placement transition among antipsychotic new users and nonusers.

	New Users	Nonusers
Descriptive Measures		
Percent of youth who experienced the first placement transition in the follow up	36.9	35.7
Mean (SD) time to the first placement transition during 180-day follow-up (days)*	109 $\pm$ 48	113 $\pm$ 54
Time to Event Measure	HR	95% CI
Likelihood of a placement transition following antipsychotic initiation	1.1	0.7–1.6

*Among youth who had any placement transition in the follow up period. The follow up period was from day 31st through day 210th after the index date.

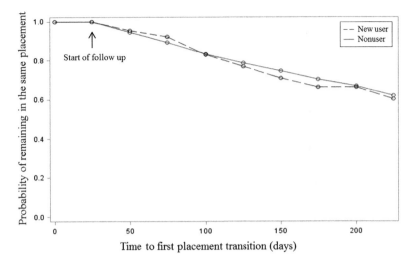

Number of youth remaining in the same foster care placement during the follow-up period*

Time(days)	0-25	25-50	50-75	75-100	100-125	125-150	150-175	175-200	200-225
New users	65	65	62	60	54	50	46	43	22.5
Nonusers	325	325	307	290	271	256	243	229	112.5

*The follow-up period starts at day 31th after the index date.

Figure 2. Kaplan-Meier estimates of foster care placement transition among new antipsychotic users and nonusers during the 180-day follow-up.

probability of staying in the same placement was higher in new users than nonuser, but the difference was not statistically significant.

The hazard ratio (HR = 1.1; 95% CI = 0.7 – 1.6) also demonstrated no difference in the likelihood of the first placement transition between new users and nonusers. The sensitivity analyses that extended the pre-index date look-back period to define a new user produced similar findings (data not shown).

Discussion

To our knowledge, this is the first observational study to integrate data from two child-serving agencies – child welfare and Medicaid – to examine the association between antipsychotic initiation and placement transition among youth with ADHD/DBD. In this study, youth who initiated antipsychotics had a similar number of placement transitions during the study follow up relative to propensity score matched nonusers. What's more, nearly two thirds of youth had no other psychotropic medications in the 180-days preceding antipsychotic initiation; this finding suggests that antipsychotics were not prescribed for adjunctive treatment as the clinical guidelines recommend for youth with ADHD/DBD (Pappadopulos et al., 2003).

Antipsychotic initiation among youth in foster care with ADHD/DBD has key public health and clinical implications. For one, antipsychotics do not have an FDA-approved indication for ADHD/DBD and few randomized controlled trials provide evidence for the efficacy of risperidone in reducing symptoms of disruptive behavior disorders (Armenteros, Lewis, & Davalos, 2007; Buitelaar, van der Gaag, Cohen-Kettenis, & Melman, 2001; Findling, 2008; Pandina, Aman, & Findling, 2006; Turgay, Binder, Snyder, & Fisman, 2002). There was only modest improvement in the children's aggressive scale (CAS) when risperidone was used in combination with stimulants for aggressive behaviors among children with ADHD, and the non-significant interaction between the CAS score and treatment groups over time suggests limited long-term benefits of risperidone (Armenteros et al., 2007). Another placebo-controlled trial among youth with conduct disorders found risperidone was superior to placebo in ameliorating aggressive behaviors in youth. However, the trial excluded youth who had moderate to severe ADHD with significant psychiatric comorbidity, and thus limiting generalizability for youth in foster care who generally have more complicated mental health issues (Findling et al., 2000).

A large number of new antipsychotic users were excluded from the sample after propensity score matching because there was no comparable control given the observed covariates. It is important to investigate those new users who failed to match on appropriate nonusers. Comparing propensity matched new users ($n = 65$) with the unmatched new users ($n = 224$) who were excluded from the study cohort, the unmatched new users were:

- younger (aged 11 years old and younger: 15.4% in matched new users vs. 44.2% in unmatched new users),
- had more internalizing disorders (40.0% in matched new users vs. 56.3% in unmatched new users), and
- fewer received psychotherapy prior to antipsychotic initiation (13.9% in matched new users vs. 3.1% in unmatched new users).

In addition to the different clinical baseline, the unmatched new users had:

- more hospitalizations (15.4% in matched new users vs. 66.1% in unmatched new users),
- emergency department visits (6.2% in matched new users vs. 16.1% in unmatched new users), and
- placement transitions prior to antipsychotic initiation (35.4% in matched new users vs. 60.1% in unmatched new users).

Data are presented in Table 3. Such patterns suggest that the study findings would not be generalizable to youth who had a more severe impairment relative to the study sample, and for whom more intensive services may be needed and placement may be less stable. For example, coordinated care using wraparound practice model has been used to provide a team-based child-center treatment plans among youth with severe emotional and behavioral disorders (Bruns & Walker, 2010; Bruns et al., 2010). Unlike standard mental health services in community-based settings, this care model has demonstrated improvements in

Table 3. Characteristics among propensity score matched and unmatched new antipsychotic users.

	Matched New Users N = 65		Unmatched New Users N = 224		
	N	%	N	%	p value
Demographic characteristics					
Age (mean, SD)	14.6 (4.0)		11.15 (4.2)		
Age (yrs)					<.05
≤5	2	3.1	24	10.7	
6–10	8	12.3	75	33.5	
11–15	23	35.4	84	37.5	
16–21	32	49.2	41	18.3	
Gender					0.607
Male	33	50.8	130	58.0	
Female	32	49.2	94	42.0	
Race					0.705
White	15	23.1	59	26.3	
Black/African American	48	73.9	160	71.4	
Others	1	1.5	4	1.8	
Clinical Characteristics					
Psychiatric diagnosis					
Externalizing disorders	65	100.0	224	100.0	
Internalizing disorders	26	40.0	126	56.3	<.001
Developmental disorders	2	3.1	14	6.3	<.05
Psychotherapy	9	13.9	7	3.1	<.05
Service Utilization					
Any hospitalization	10	15.4	148	66.1	<.05
Any emergency department visit	4	6.2	36	16.1	<.001
Any placement transition	23	35.4	136	60.7	<.05

reduction of numbers of school suspensions, out of home placements, inpatient psychiatric hospital admissions, and medical costs (Wraparound Milwaukee-2012 Year End report.2012; CHIPRA Quality Demonstration Grant Program Webinar Series, 2013; Louisiana Behavioral Health Partnership, 2013). The association between antipsychotic initiation and placement stability is worthy of future investigation to determine the effect of care coordination on antipsychotic prescribing for youth with severe behavioral disorders.

The study is not without limitations. First, as noted previously, the results could only be applicable to youth who had demographic and clinical profiles similar to that of the study sample. The findings may not be generalizable to youth in other settings where clinical practice and state-level regulations for antipsychotics monitoring may differ. Second, placement transitions for this study were conceptualized as movement to any other placement; either a less restrictive (e.g., a child was moved from a residential treatment center to foster home) or more restrictive situation (e.g., a child was moved from a group home to residential treatment center). The type of placement transition could influence medication use. For example, a less restrictive, more home-based placement transition might lead to improvement in better management of behavior and, therefore, less need for medication. There are no studies we are aware of that examine the association between the restrictiveness of placement and psychotropic initiation. Furthermore, some placement changes may be clinically beneficial to the youth, and this study could not determine the appropriateness of the transition. Third, it was not possible to assess disease severity, which is a limitation common to all administrative data. This study attempted to minimize this bias by applying propensity score methods and restricting the sample to youth with ADHD/DBD in the absence of more severe mental health disorders such as schizophrenia and bipolar disorders. Although other factors such as foster family characteristics and proxies for clinical status, such as laboratory results, might improve propensity score matching, these are unobserved covariates in the claims-based observational study. Fourth, it is acknowledged that individual antipsychotic agents have different benefit-risk profiles for managing disruptive behavior disorders in youth (Pringsheim & Gorman, 2012); however, the small sample available in this analysis prohibited subgroup analysis. Finally, claims-based ICD-9 diagnosis codes are limited in that investigators are not able to validate this against a formal clinical evaluation.

Despite the limitations, this study has two important strengths. First, linked data from two child-serving agencies provided an enriched examination of the association between antipsychotic initiation and risk of placement transition among youth in foster care with ADHD/DBD. Second, this study utilized a new user design, which is a rigorous methodological design to avoid prevalence bias that could alter the interpretation of the effect of antipsychotic use on placement stability. Youth who have been using antipsychotics (i.e., prevalent users) may have overcome treatment "failures," and are now in a more stable setting.

Conclusion

Pharmacologic interventions may be necessary but not sufficient to manage behavioral disorders given the complicated clinical and social circumstances of youth in foster care. The findings can be used to inform healthcare professionals and policymakers of the variability in the need for mental health services among youth initiating treatment with an antipsychotic. Further study is needed to assess the impact of a child-centered comprehensive treatment plan, which involves input from the child, the child's foster family members, healthcare professionals, school personnel, and caseworkers, on reducing antipsychotic use and on enhancing foster placement stability.

Funding

This project is sponsored by the Department of Health and Mental Hygiene, the Mental Hygiene Administration via the 1915(c) Home and Community-Based Waiver Program Management, Workforce Development and Evaluation (OPASS# 13-10954G/M00B3400369).

References

Armenteros, J. L., Lewis, J. E., & Davalos, M. (2007). Risperidone augmentation for treatment-resistant aggression in attention-deficit/hyperactivity disorder: A placebo-controlled pilot study. *Journal of the American Academy of Child and Adolescent Psychiatry, 46*(5), 558–565.

Barber, J. G., Delfabbro, P. H., & Cooper, L. L. (2001). The predictors of unsuccessful transition to foster care. *Journal of Child Psychology and Psychiatry, and Allied Disciplines, 42*(6), 785–790.

Bruns, E. J., & Walker, J. S. (2010). Defining practice: Flexibility, legitimacy, and the nature of systems of care and Wraparound. *Evaluation and Program Planning, 33*(1), 45–48.

Bruns, E. J., Walker, J. S., Zabel, M., Matarese, M., Estep, K., Harburger, D., & Pires, S. A. (2010). Intervening in the lives of youth with complex behavioral health challenges and their families: The role of the Wraparound process. *American Journal of Community Psychology, 46*(3–4), 314–331.

Buitelaar, J. K., van der Gaag, R. J., Cohen-Kettenis, P., & Melman, C. T. (2001). A randomized controlled trial of risperidone in the treatment of aggression in hospitalized adolescents with subaverage cognitive abilities. *Journal of Clinical Psychiatry, 62*(4), 239–248.

Carnochan, S., Moore, M., & Austin, M. J. (2013). Achieving placement stability. *Journal of Evidence-Based Social Work, 10*(3), 235–253.

CHIPRA Quality Demonstration Grant Program Webinar Series. (2013). *Improving behavioral health care quality for children and adolescents: Section of Maryland/Georgia/Wyoming— Using Care Management Entities.* Retrieved from https://www.medicaid.gov/medicaid-chip-program-information/by-topics/childrens-health-insurance-program-chip/downloads/chipra-quality-demos-webinar-1.pdf

Cooper, W. O., Arbogast, P. G., Ding, H., Hickson, G. B., Fuchs, D. C., & Ray, W. A. (2006). Trends in prescribing of antipsychotic medications for US children. *Ambulatory Pediatrics, 6*(2), 79–83.

Cooper, W. O., Hickson, G. B., Fuchs, C., Arbogast, P. G., & Ray, W. A. (2004). New users of antipsychotic medications among children enrolled in TennCare. *Archives of Pediatrics & Adolescent Medicine, 158*(8), 753–759.

Crystal, S., Olfson, M., Huang, C., Pincus, H., & Gerhard, T. (2009a). Broadened use of atypical antipsychotics: Safety, effectiveness, and policy challenges. *Health Affairs (Project Hope), 28*(5), w770–81.

Crystal, S., Olfson, M., Huang, C., Pincus, H., & Gerhard, T. (2009b). Broadened use of atypical antipsychotics: Safety, effectiveness, and policy challenges. *Health Affairs (Project Hope), 28*(5), w770–81.

dosReis, S., Yoon, Y., Rubin, D. M., Riddle, M. A., Noll, E., & Rothbard, A. (2011). Antipsychotic treatment among youth in foster care. *Pediatrics, 128*(6), e1459–1466.

Findling, R. L. (2008). Atypical antipsychotic treatment of disruptive behavior disorders in children and adolescents. *Journal of Clinical Psychiatry, 69*(Suppl 4), 9–14.

Findling, R. L., McNamara, N. K., Branicky, L. A., Schluchter, M. D., Lemon, E., & Blumer, J. L. (2000). A double-blind pilot study of risperidone in the treatment of conduct disorder. *Journal of the American Academy of Child and Adolescent Psychiatry, 39*(4), 509–516.

Fisher, P. A., Stoolmiller, M., Mannering, A. M., Takahashi, A., & Chamberlain, P. (2011). Foster placement disruptions associated with problem behavior: Mitigating a threshold effect. *Journal of Consulting and Clinical Psychology, 79*(4), 481–487.

John, M. Eisenberg Center for Clinical Decisions and Communications Science. (2007). Off-label use of atypical antipsychotics: An update. *Comparative Effectiveness Review Summary Guides for Clinicians.*

Johnson, C., Silver, P., & Wulczyn, F. (2013). *Raising the bar for health and mental health services for children in foster care: Developing a model of managed care.* Council of Family and Child Caring Agencies and New York State Health Foundation. Retrieved from http://www.cofcca.org/pdfs/FosterCareManagedCare-FinalReport.pdf

Jonson-Reid, M., & Barth, R. P. (2000). From maltreatment report to juvenile incarceration: The role of child welfare services. *Child Abuse & Neglect, 24*(4), 505–520.

Leathers, S. J. (2006). Placement disruption and negative placement outcomes among adolescents in long-term foster care: The role of behavior problems. *Child Abuse & Neglect, 30*(3), 307–324.

Louisiana Behavioral Health Partnership. (2013). *Coordinated system of care (CSoC)–transforming the system.* Retrieved from http://dhh.louisiana.gov/index.cfm/page/454/n/180

Loy, J. H., Merry, S. N., Hetrick, S. E., & Stasiak, K. (2012). Atypical antipsychotics for disruptive behaviour disorders in children and youths. *The Cochrane Database of Systematic Reviews, 9,* CD008559.

Maglione, M., Ruelaz Maher, A., Hu, J., Wang, Z., Shanman, R., Shekelle, P. G., Roth, B., Hilton, L., Suttorp, M. J., Ewing, B. A., Motala, A., Perry, T. (2011). *Off-label use of atypical antipsychotics: an update. Comparative Effectiveness Review No. 43.* (Prepared by the Southern California Evidence-based Practice Center under Contract No. HHSA290-2007-10062-1). Rockville, MD: Agency for Healthcare Research and Quality. Retrieved from http://www.effectivehealthcare.ahrq.gov/reports/final.cfm

Newton, R. R., Litrownik, A. J., & Landsverk, J. A. (2000). Children and youth in foster care: Disentangling the relationship between problem behaviors and number of placements. *Child Abuse & Neglect, 24*(10), 1363–1374.

Olfson, M., Blanco, C., Liu, L., Moreno, C., & Laje, G. (2006). National trends in the outpatient treatment of children and adolescents with antipsychotic drugs. *Archives of General Psychiatry, 63*(6), 679–685.

Olfson, M., Blanco, C., Liu, S. M., Wang, S., & Correll, C. U. (2012). National trends in the office-based treatment of children, adolescents, and adults with antipsychotics. *Archives of General Psychiatry, 69*(12), 1247–1256.

Pandina, G. J., Aman, M. G., & Findling, R. L. (2006). Risperidone in the management of disruptive behavior disorders. *Journal of Child and Adolescent Psychopharmacology, 16*(4), 379–392.

Pappadopulos, E., Macintyre Ii, J. C., Crismon, M. L., Findling, R. L., Malone, R. P., Derivan, A., & Jensen, P. S. (2003). Treatment recommendations for the use of antipsychotics for aggressive youth (TRAAY): Part II. *Journal of the American Academy of Child and Adolescent Psychiatry, 42*(2), 145–161.

Parsons, L. (2004). *Performing a 1:N case-control match on propensity score.* Retrieved from http://www2.sas.com/proceedings/sugi29/165–29.pdf

Pringsheim, T., & Gorman, D. (2012). Second-generation antipsychotics for the treatment of disruptive behaviour disorders in children: A systematic review. *Canadian Journal of Psychiatry/Revue Canadienne De Psychiatrie, 57*(12), 722–727.

Rubin, D. M., Feudtner, C., Localio, R., & Mandell, D. S. (2009). State variation in psychotropic medication use by foster care children with autism spectrum disorder. *Pediatrics, 124*(2), e305–12.

Rubin, D. M., O'Reilly, A. L., Luan, X., & Localio, A. R. (2007). The impact of placement stability on behavioral well-being for children in foster care. *Pediatrics, 119*(2), 336–344.

Taber, M. A., & Proch, K. (1987). Placement stability for adolescents in foster care: Findings from a program experiment. *Child Welfare, 66*(5), 433–445.

University of California Davis Extension, The Center for Human Services. (2008). *A literature review of placement stability in child welfare service: Issues, concerns, outcomes and future directions*. Retrieved from http://www.childsworld.ca.gov/res/pdf/PlacementStability.pdf

Turgay, A., Binder, C., Snyder, R., & Fisman, S. (2002). Long-term safety and efficacy of risperidone for the treatment of disruptive behavior disorders in children with subaverage IQs. *Pediatrics, 110*(3), e34.

U.S. Department of Health and Human Services, Administration for Children and Families, Administration on Children, Youth and Families, Children's Bureau. (2014). *The AFCARS report*. Retrieved from http://www.acf.hhs.gov/sites/default/files/cb/afcarsreport19.pdf

Wraparound Milwaukee. (2012). *Wraparound Milwaukee- 2012 Year End Report*. Retrieved from http://wraparoundmke.com/wp-content/uploads/2013/11/WMAnnualReport_2012.pdf

Zhou, Z., Rahme, E., Abrahamowicz, M., & Pilote, L. (2005). Survival bias associated with time-to-treatment initiation in drug effectiveness evaluation: A comparison of methods. *American Journal of Epidemiology, 162*(10), 1016–1023.

Zito, J. M., Burcu, M., Ibe, A., Safer, D. J., & Magder, L. S. (2013). Antipsychotic use by Medicaid-insured youths: Impact of eligibility and psychiatric diagnosis across a decade. *Psychiatric Services (Washington, DC), 64*(3), 223–229.

From Maltreatment to Delinquency: Service Trajectories After a First Intervention of Child Protection Services

Catherine Laurier, Sonia Hélie, Catherine Pineau-Villeneuve, and Marie-Noële Royer

ABSTRACT
The relationship between maltreatment in childhood and delinquency in adolescence is recognized. However, the data available do not reveal what proportion of children under the supervision of child protection services (CPS) later transfer to youth legal services, nor the sequence of services provided by these two systems. This study sketches a preliminary portrait of Youth Criminal Justice Act (YCJA) incidence among Quebec children and adolescents as a consequence of a first crime after initial CPS case closure (N = 14,252). It quantifies the scope of the phenomenon and identifies the best predictors of YCJA incidence from among the administrative data available. Survival analysis revealed a 15.4% YCJA incidence for the entire cohort in the five and a half years following termination of initial intervention; boys between 12 and 17 years old when their initial CPS cases were closed were at the greatest risk (27.2%).

Prior work on the risk of juvenile-justice-system entry among children receiving child protection services (CPS) has documented the scope of the crossover between the two systems and the factors associated with it. These studies indicate that the presence of behavior problems in youth, as assessed by researchers for research purposes, followed by CPS is a strong determinant of later delinquency. In the Province of Quebec, the law that regulates the provision of CPS (Youth Protection Act—YPA) stipulates that serious behavioral problems in a youth are sufficient grounds to justify the intervention of CPS. This specificity is also reflected in the manner of recording administrative data on child maltreatment and juvenile delinquency, so that the study of the pathway from maltreatment to delinquency is facilitated by an integrated client-information system. The aim of this article is to examine the incidence of youth criminal justice entry after CPS closure in this unique context in which children in need of protection because of their behavior can be formally taken care of under these grounds. Before reviewing the literature on the frequency and risk factors of juvenile justice entry among children followed by CPS, an overview of the legislative and organizational context that prevails in Quebec is proposed.

Legislative and organizational context

Under Canada's constitution, the provinces are responsible for administering child protection laws and systems. In Quebec, Section 38 of the Youth Protection Act (YPA; 2009) defines the circumstances in which children's safety or development are deemed to be endangered and the remedial measures that may be taken. The YPA may be enforced on a number of grounds: abandonment [paragraph 38(a)], neglect [paragraph 38(b)], psychological maltreatment [paragraph 38(c)], sexual abuse [paragraph 38(d)], physical abuse [paragraph 38(e)], and serious behavioral disturbance [paragraph 38(f)]. When we began the study under discussion in 2009, Quebec CPS agencies had registered a total of 30,022 investigated reports (2009). Those reports concerned 25,437 children (some were reported more than once in the same year). Eighty-four percent of children receiving postinvestigation services were protected due to some form of maltreatment, while 16% received CPS for their serious behavior problems (Association des Centres jeunesse du Québec, 2015).

Unlike similar laws in other jurisdictions, the YPA recognizes serious behavioral disturbance as a type of child endangerment and grounds for intervention. These disturbances are defined as follows in the YPA:

> [The term] "serious behavioral disturbance" refers to a situation in which a child behaves in such a way as to repeatedly or seriously undermine the child's or others' physical or psychological integrity, and the child's parents fail to take the necessary steps to put an end to the situation or, if the child is 14 or over, the child objects to such steps. (Paragraph 38f)

Specifically, it may be behaviors that are detrimental to others, such as aggressions, bullying, or behaviors wherein the youth puts himself or herself in danger, such as suicidal tendencies, self-mutilation, or the abuse of drugs or alcohol (Ministry of Health and Social Services, 2010).

Some studies indicate that certain protection systems take the problematic behavior of their users into account (Dandreaux & Frick, 2009; Ryan, 2012; Wright, McMahon, Daly, & Haney, 2012). However, these problem behaviors are detected after entering protective services on the grounds of maltreatment. This characteristic of the Quebec legislation of including serious behavioral problems as grounds for protection allows for intervention directly toward the child's behavioral problems, both to protect the child and keep him or her from a path of delinquency.

The Youth Criminal Justice Act (YCJA; 2009) applies to youths between 12 and 17 years of age who have violated the Criminal Code or committed other federal crimes (2009). The YCJA's goal is to protect the public, prevent crime, foster responsibility, and promote rehabilitation and reintegration. In 2008–2009, 15,751 young offenders under the YCJA received services. That year, a total of 3,723 youths were given 5,214 sentences under the YCJA (mean of 1.4 sentences per youth). As of March 31, 2009, 80% of the clients served by the agency (Montreal's CPS agency) were children receiving services under the YPA, 13% were adolescents receiving services under the YCJA, and 2% were adolescents receiving services under both acts (2009). The rest were receiving general social services under the Act Respecting Health Services and Social Services. However, data available at present for Quebec do not reveal what proportion of children under the supervision of CPS later transfer to youth criminal justice services, nor the sequence of the two types of services. A number of local authors suggest that for most adolescents dealt with under the YCJA, it is not their first contact with the system (Moreau, 2007; Pauzé et al., 2004; Tourigny et al., 2002). In fact, a good many of them have already experienced a CPS intervention on a variety of endangerment grounds.

Juvenile delinquency among children followed by CPS

Among youth under the care of CPS, age is a major risk factor for delinquency. Until recently, a consensus had begun to emerge in the literature to the effect that early exposure to abuse greatly increased the likelihood of developmental problems. However, recent studies show that the greater the age before the first intervention, the more the child or youth is likely to engage in delinquent behavior (Goodkind, Shook, Kim, Pohlig, & Herring, 2013; Verrecchia, Fetzer, Lemmon, & Austin, 2010). Moreover, a recent U.S. study contends that in children aged 7 to 17 years who were subject to an intervention by Florida welfare services ($N = 13,212$), each additional year before the intervention increases the risk of migrating toward youth criminal justice services by 47% (Yampolskaya, Armstrong, & McNeish, 2011). This means that the earlier CPS intervenes, the more likely youth delinquency can be prevented.

A number of authors have examined the relationship between age and delinquency (including Farrington, 1986; Fréchette & Le Blanc, 1987; Moffitt & Caspi, 2001). It has thus been demonstrated many times over that early behavioral problems are predictors of aggravation and diversification of future delinquency (Craig, Petrunka, & Khan, 2011; Fréchette & Le Blanc, 1987; Moffitt & Caspi, 2001). In fact, longitudinal studies have shown it to be unlikely that an adolescent who has never been aggressive before would suddenly begin to display serious behavioral problems and aggressiveness (Tremblay, 2012). According to developmental criminology, violent delinquency is linked to aggressive behavior already present in childhood (Farrington, 1986; Fortin & Strayer, 2000).

It is generally agreed that boys and girls show different patterns of delinquency (Cernkovich, Kaukinen, & Giordano, 2005; Lanctôt & Le Blanc, 2002). Being a boy is certainly one of the risk factors for delinquency most cited in the literature (Chiu, Ryan, & Herz, 2011). Although the sex of the child or youth is not associated with CPS intervention, boys are overrepresented in the juvenile justice system (Goodkind et al., 2013; Puzzanchera, Adams, & Sickmund, 2010). A number of studies have demonstrated that there are fairly large differences between boys and girls with regard to the type, duration, and seriousness of their delinquency (Cernkovich et al., 2005; Côté, Tremblay, & Vitaro, 2003; Lanctôt & Le Blanc, 2002; Sprott, Doob, & Jenkins, 2001, among others). According to Moffitt and Caspi (2001), the ratios of boys and girls following different (adolescence-limited or severe and persistent) antisocial pathways are not the same, either. They found a male-to-female ratio of 10:1 for severe and persistent childhood-onset delinquency but only 1.5:1 for adolescence-onset delinquency (Moffitt & Caspi, 2001). Some researchers have found that sex differences in delinquency are attributable to the different ways boys and girls are affected by risk and protective factors (Fitzgerald, 2003). For example, girls appear to be more sensitive than boys to the effects of family violence (Bender, 2010).

Similarly, Tourigny et al. (2002) have shown that boys and girls are not reported to CPS nor in the same proportion. Girls are primarily reported for neglect, followed by behavioral problems, while for boys, it is the opposite. In addition, the few descriptive studies done in Quebec, surveyed by Moreau (2007), cover services received by children under the YPA. These studies clearly demonstrate the differences between the sexes in terms of grounds for reporting, age at time of receiving services, and types of measures taken. Boys and girls also seem to manifest their adjustment problems differently. Girls are more prone to internalizing symptoms, such as anxiety disorders or depression, along with self-risk behaviors, such as belonging to antisocial groups (Lanctôt & Desaive, 2002). Most boys, on the other hand, exhibit externalized and aggressive behaviors, such as delinquency (Lanctôt & Desaive, 2002; Lanctôt & Le Blanc, 2002; Tourigny et al., 2002). This suggests that the risks of girls and boys receiving an extrajudicial sanction or a judicial measure under the YCJA (which we will call a "YCJA event") may also be different.

Maltreatment during childhood has, for years, been included in the etiology of delinquency; that is to say, it has been observed that a history of physical, sexual, or psychological abuse, and emotional and physical negligence, all increase the likelihood of offending behavior (Bender, 2010; Crooks, Scott, Wolfe, Chiodo, & Killip, 2007; Ryan & Testa, 2005; Verrecchia et al., 2010). This effect has been consistently documented in meta-analyzes (Derzon, 2010). The authors report prevalence of maltreatment ranging from 26% to 60% among young people supported by the youth criminal justice system (Bender, 2010; Currie & Tekin, 2011; Ford, Hartman, Hawke, & Chapman, 2008; Lemmon, 2006; Mallett, 2014; Sedlak & McPherson, 2010; Stouthamer-Loeber, Loeber, Wei, Farrington, & Wikström, 2002). Although the presence of maltreatment history is high among these young people, note however that the majority of maltreated children and adolescents will not become offenders (Widom, 2003; Yun, Ball, & Lim, 2011). Furthermore, the literature is clear about the chronicity of maltreatment. Thus, regardless of the type, it is an important risk factor both in the initiation, continuation, and worsening of delinquency (Lemmon, 2006; Verrecchia et al., 2010; Yun et al., 2011). Moreover, young people who began to suffer maltreatment in childhood that continued through adolescence are more at risk of offending than those who suffered maltreatment mostly in childhood (Stewart, Livingston, & Dennison, 2008). This relationship continues to be important even when adding other risk factors such as gender, socioeconomic status, or place of residence (Ireland, Smith, & Thornberry, 2002; Van Wert, Ma, Lefebvre, & Fallon, 2013).

In addition, it appears that most of the behaviors that lead to care under the YPA due to behavioral problems are relatively well-accepted risk factors in the literature. This is particularly the case for antisocial behavior and behavioral problems that include a wide range of conduct, including criminal offenses, drug and alcohol use, risky sexual behavior and aggression (Hawkins et al., 2000). For example, Case & Haines (2007) found that antisocial attitudes and behaviors are among the most important risk factors for delinquency regardless of gender, type of offense, or age group. Many authors agree that general delinquency such as theft, vandalism, or violence toward others is an indicator of subsequent delinquency (Gatti, Tremblay, & Vitaro, 2009; Shader, 2003). This means that there could be chronic disruptive behaviors that evolve and worsen to become real delinquent and criminal behaviors (Lipsey & Derzon, 1998).

Many authors have come to different conclusions when it comes to measuring the impact of CPS intervention on the development of delinquent behaviors (DeGue & Widom, 2009; Goodkind et al., 2013; Lemmon, 2006). Jonson-Reid (2002) found that children with a CPS intervention who receive services at home are less at risk of offending than those who do not receive services or who are placed in substitute care. Baskins and Sommers (2011) found no difference in the type of intervention on delinquency. Still others found that children placed in substitute care by CPS have a higher prevalence of violent and delinquent behaviors and of developmental problems than those who remain in their home during CPS intervention (Ford et al., 2010; Keil & Price, 2006; Maschi, Hatcher, Schwalbe, & Rosato, 2008). However, very few studies have examined the different characteristics of the intervention apart from the presence of substitute care placement.

In addition, Ryan (2012) stressed that no study to date has been able to consider CPS intervention on any other grounds than maltreatment. In his study, he hypothesizes that youth placed in substitute care by CPS who also have behavioral disorders would be more likely to migrate to the U.S. juvenile criminal system because CPS is not adapted to this type of clientele. The recommended interventions will therefore not be able to put a stop to the development of delinquent behavior. In addition, youths placed in substitute care by CPS who also present disruptive behaviors are more likely to be moved from one placement setting to another (Keil & Price, 2006; Leathers, 2006) and will be in care longer than those without behavioral problems (Baskins &

Sommers, 2011). In addition, the instability of placement and duration of services provided by CPS contribute to delinquency risk factors (Ryan & Testa, 2005). Indeed, researchers associate this placement instability to increased risk of entering the youth criminal justice system (DeGue & Widom, 2009; Goodkind et al., 2013; Jonson-Reid & Barth, 2000b). However, no one has been able to demonstrate that it is actually the instability that increases the risk of delinquency or if, conversely, it is youths who already present early problem behaviors who are more likely to experience placement instability (Newton, Litrownik, & Landsverk, 2000; Ryan & Testa, 2005).

Aim of the current study

YCJA incidence after one or more reports to CPS deserves special attention. Although a number of studies have suggested that maltreatment in childhood contributes in various ways to delinquency in adolescence, none has specifically estimated the risk of a juvenile criminal services entry or tried to understand the sequence of events between first receipt of CPS and first legal sanction in a context in which CPS can intervene formally and explicitly on the behavior problems exhibited by a youth. It is important to gain a better understanding of the factors most likely to influence the risk of evolving from a child in need of protection to perpetrator among youth who first receive services as a result of maltreatment or serious behavioral disturbance. Better knowledge of these mechanisms will enable us to adapt services to the children and adolescents at greatest risk of delinquency.

In this study, juvenile delinquency is conceptualized as a multidimensional phenomenon that is influenced by complex interactions between individual, family, and environmental factors. In that sense, our work can be seen as adopting Bronfenbrenner's ecological model of human development (Bronfenbrenner, 1979). In accordance with this conceptual framework, we tried, as much as possible, to introduce in our analysis variables, among those available in the data set, that cover different ecosystems constituting the situation of a child exiting CPS.

The overall objective of this study is to assess YCJA incidence after initial CPS case closure and to identify associated factors in the specific context of Quebec wherein a youth can receive CPS solely on the grounds of exhibiting serious behavioral problems.

Method

Background and data sources

In Quebec, CPS agencies are responsible for enforcing the YPA and offering services to children in difficulty and to their families, including services to young offenders followed under the YCJA. To establish a province-wide representative profile and for feasibility's sake, the Quebec clinical/ administrative databases were the only data sources used. These data sets integrate administrative data regarding CPS provided as well as services provided under the YCJA. Since 2003, all 16 CPS agencies in Quebec have been using the same management information system to track their clients and store information about situations reported, the children's characteristics, and services provided. The data entered into the system are standardized throughout all the agencies and cross-checked for reliability.

Cohort under study

During the study's 5-year eligibility period (January 1, 2005, to December 31, 2009), 25,897 children received postinvestigation services from Quebec CPS agencies. Postinvestigation services include a variety of protective measures that take the form, for example, of a placement in substitute care or psychosocial support. Note that the CPS can be offered on a voluntary basis (not judicialized) or by going to court (judicialized). A total of 18,439 of the children receiving postinvestigation services during the targeted period were at risk of a YCJA event because they turned 12 before the end of the observation period (June 30, 2010). However, 3,742 of them had their initial CPS cases closed on their 18th birthday; in other words, they aged out of the system. They were therefore at no risk of a YCJA event *after* initial CPS case closure, so they were eliminated from the sample. Another 445 children committed their first offenses while still receiving postinvestigation services. As the subject of this study is the risk of a YCJA event occurring *after* initial CPS case closure, they were also eliminated for two reasons. First, children with an active file under the YPA may be subject to a surveillance bias, since they are more exposed to the expert eyes of CPS workers. Including these cases in the sample would result in an overestimation of the risk of an incident under the YCJA after CPS closure. Second, we wanted to focus on the more problematic cases in which CPS intervention had come to an end, meaning that protection measures were applied and the security/development of the child was judged to no longer be endangered, and in which there was a subsequent event reported under the YCJA. The final cohort studied was therefore made up of 14,252 adolescents whose initial cases were closed between 2005 and 2009 and were at risk of committing a first offense leading to extrajudicial sanctions or measures under the YCJA during the observation period. Children were followed from CPS closure to June 30, 2010. The length of follow-up thus varies from 6 months to 5.5 years, depending on the date of entry into the cohort.

It is important to note that two areas in northern Quebec are not included in the study, because child protection services are not provided by dedicated agencies but by local community service centers (CLSCs), which do not use the same management information system. A mere 0.8% of the children in the province live there. Thus, the cohort under study comprised all the children, whether of Aboriginal descent or not, served by Quebec 16 CPS agencies.

Variables

We have defined a *YCJA event* as the application of any extrajudicial sanction or judicial measure under the YCJA as a consequence of a first offense committed after initial CPS case closure. An offense alone therefore does not constitute a YCJA event; an extrajudicial sanction or judicial measure must have been imposed. Services counted as YCJA events are "supervision of extrajudicial sanctions," "supervision of sentences," and "presentence supervision." This decision was made in order to ensure that only offenses for which the adolescent was found guilty were considered. (If there was no extrajudicial sanction or judicial measure, either the adolescent was found not guilty or the offense was deemed minor.)

The YCJA event date is the date the offense was committed. The commission of an offense triggered the YCJA event. When more than one offense was committed at the same time, they were grouped and the penalties and sentences were imposed for the multiple offenses. We analyzed *YCJA incidence*, or risk of occurrence of a YCJA event, in relation to a series of factors to identify the best predictors. The factors can be divided into two categories: the child's characteristics and those of the initial postinvestigation services.

The child's characteristics in the database are as follows: age, sex, and Aboriginal descent. The child's *age* is defined in three different ways, depending on the type of analysis: age at time of report leading to initial postinvestigation services, age at time of YCJA event, or age at start of observation period (or initial case closure). The child's *sex* is also taken into account. Lastly, *Aboriginal descent* includes Indians living on and off reserve, and Aboriginal people recognized under the James Bay and Northern Quebec Agreement, Inuit, and Métis.

The variables associated with the characteristics of initial postinvestigation services were grounds for intervention, duration of services, court involvement, out-of-home placement, CPS recurrence, discontinuity, and CPS history. The *grounds for intervention* were the reasons for providing protective services, as recorded at the end of the initial assessment. Possible grounds were neglect, physical abuse, sexual abuse, serious behavioral disturbance, and abandonment. The primary grounds for postinvestigation services were used either alone or in addition to secondary grounds, as needed for the analyses. *Duration of services* is the number of days from the date the initial report was received until the initial case was closed. *Court involvement* is when a CPS case is brought before the court, either because there was no agreement on the intervention plan or because of the seriousness of the case. *Placement* means that the child was removed from the family home at least once between receipt of the initial report and case closure. Placement could be accommodation in a CPS facility or with a significant person. *CPS recurrence* is defined as an investigated and substantiated report after initial case closure and within the observation period. *Discontinuity* means that more than one caseworker per year was assigned during the initial services. Depending on the analysis, *CPS history* may include reports prior to the initial report, either investigated or not.

Analytical framework

Survival analysis is the analytical method selected for this study. It allowed us to estimate YCJA incidence over a period of 5.5 years, while at the same time taking into account unequal observation periods and adolescents who aged out of the system within the observation period. The relative risk considers both whether or not there was a YCJA offense and the cumulative time that each child was at risk of a YCJA event, but did not experience it (survival time). For the children without a YCJA event, survival time is the number of days between initial case closure and the end of the observation period (June 30, 2009) or their 18th birthday, whichever came first. For the rest, survival time is the number of days between initial case closure and the date of the YCJA event. For children not yet 12 years old at initial case closure who turned 12 within the observation period (minimum age to be at risk of a YCJA event), survival time is the time between their 12th birthday and the occurrence of the YCJA event or the end of the observation period, whichever came first.

Two sets of analyses were done to assess YCJA incidence in the cohort under study. After estimating the cohort's YCJA incidence using survival analysis (Kaplan-Meier model), we performed multivariate regression analyses (Cox regressions) to identify which of the characteristics of the children and the initial services in the database were the best predictors. Investigations for possible multicollinearity revealed that there were no multicollinearity problems among the covariates in any of the age groups. The variance inflating factors were under the critical value of 5, as recommended by Tabachnick and Fidell (2013) for all covariates.

Results

Description of cohort

Table 1 describes the main characteristics of the cohort under study. Age at time of initial report is fairly high in our cohort, compared with the age of all children under CPS supervision, since the children in the sample had to be at risk of a YCJA event by December 30, 2009, and so had to have turned 12 by that date. The youngest therefore had to be 7 at the start of the cohort eligibility period of January 1, 2005.

Table 1. Description of cohort.

Characteristics	Cohort[a] (%)
Age at initial report (years)	
0–5	4.8
6–11	42.6
12–17	52.6
Age at start of observation period (at risk) (years)	
12 (after a delay because initial case was closed before child turned 12)	20.6
12–14	30.6
15–17	43.3
Initial reporter	
Child	1.2
Parent	12.7
Relative or acquaintance (parent's partner, sibling, relative, foster family, neighbor)	7.5
School	20.4
Police	14.3
CPS agency	10.9
CLSC	9.9
Other	23.1
Sex	
Boy	47
Girl	53
Aboriginal descent	4.6
At least one prior investigated report	90.4
Priority level of initial report	
Immediate	21
24 hours	11.9
4 days	55.6
Unknown	11.5
Primary ground for initial intervention	
Neglect (or risk thereof)	52.6
Physical abuse (or risk thereof)	9.8
Sexual abuse (or risk thereof)	5.7
Abandonment	1.3
Psychological abuse	1.8
Behavioral problems	28.8
Placement at time of initial intervention	49.7
CPS recurrence	21.7
Mean age at initial report (years)	11.3
Mean age at start of observation period (years)	14.1
Mean number of caseworkers	2.46
Mean duration of services from initial report (days)	805

[a] $N = 14,252$.

Only 4.8% of the cohort were 5 or under at the time of the initial report. (They received initial postinvestigation services for a long time but not until they aged out and would have been eliminated from the cohort, which explains why there are so few of them.) Mean age at the time of the initial report was 11.3 years. Mean age at the start of the observation period was 14.1 years, after receiving services for an average of 805 days (2.2 years). The cohort consists of slightly more boys (53%) than girls (47%). The proportion of children of Aboriginal descent is 4.6%. Although none of the children in the cohort had received postinvestigation services earlier, 90% had been the subject of one or more investigated reports.

The initial report was made most often, in close to 35% of cases, by the school or the police. CPS employees reported 11% of the children and local community services centers, 10%.

Table 1 also shows the various characteristics of the services, such as grounds for intervention, placement, and recurrence. As can be seen, more than half of children (52.6%) were under supervision on the primary grounds of neglect. The second most common issue pertained to behavioral problems, for 28.8% of the cohort. Sexual and physical abuse represented 5.7% and 9.8% of the cohort, respectively. Abandonment, an extreme form of neglect, concerned 1.3% of the children in the cohort. The 1.8% of psychological abuse seen in our cohort underestimates the true scope of this form of maltreatment, since only situations reported after July 2007 can be legally recognized as such under new provisions of the YPA that came into effect at that time. A proportion of 21.7% of the children in the cohort returned to CPS supervision after initial case closure and before the YCJA event (CPS recurrence). While receiving postinvestigation services for the first time, the children had an average of 2.5 caseworkers successively assigned to them. Lastly, 49.7% of the children in the cohort received out-of-home placements (including with a significant person).

YCJA incidence

First YCJA offense occurred an average of 461 days (1.3 years) after initial case closure or turning 12 (for those whose initial cases were closed before they turned 12). Mean age at first offense was 15, but first extrajudicial measures or legal sanctions were imposed at 15.6 years of age.

Figure 1, which concerns only adolescents who experienced a YCJA event, shows the time between initial case closure (or turning 12, for the youngest

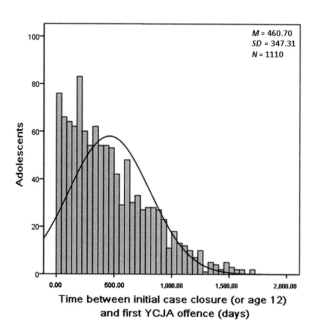

Figure 1. Time (in days) between initial case closure (or turning 12) and YCJA offense.

ones) and the first offense counted toward YCJA incidence. The positive asymmetrical curve shows that the longer the time since initial case closure, the lower the YCJA incidence.

Offences associated with first YCJA event

The type of offenses that triggered the first YCJA event varied greatly among the 1,110 adolescents who committed them, and the number of offenses ranged from 1 all the way to 83 ($M = 2.74$). Almost three adolescents out of four (73.7%) committed one or two offenses, but 3.6% of them had committed more than 10 offenses at the time of their first YCJA event. Most of the offenses related to the first YCJA event were crimes against property (55.1%), followed by crimes against persons (44%).

Survival analyses

As the survival curve in Figure 2 shows, 15.4% of children who received initial postinvestigation services had committed a YCJA offense by the end of our 5-year observation period.

Before going into further detail about the analyses to determine which factors had the greatest influence on YCJA incidence after initial case closure, it is important to look at whether the girls and boys in the cohort had the same incidence pattern. Figure 3 shows survival curves by sex.

As Figure 3 shows, boys are at much greater risk of committing a YCJA offense than girls in the 5 years following initial case closure or upon turning 12. While the 5-year incidence for girls is 7.1%, it is almost three times greater

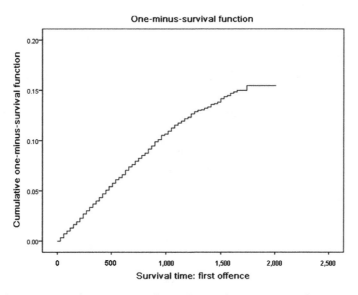

Figure 2. Risk group's cumulative YCJA incidence during observation period.

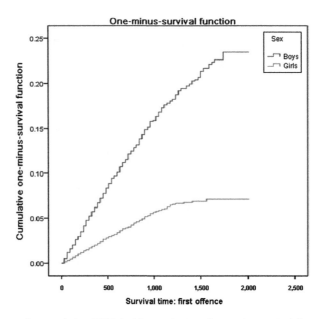

Figure 3. Risk group's cumulative YCJA incidence during observation period, by sex.

at 23.4% for boys. These findings are in line with those of the vast majority of studies on the subject (Bright & Jonson-Reid, 2008; Chiu et al., 2011; Jonson-Reid, 2002; Jonson-Reid & Barth, 2000a; Ryan & Testa, 2005). Based on this significant disparity, subsequent analyses were performed separately for boys and girls in the cohort.

As mentioned earlier, the youths in the cohort must have turned 12 by the end of the observation period to be at risk of a YCJA offense. So for those whose initial cases were closed after they turned 12, the observation period started immediately at that point. However, for those whose initial cases were closed before they turned 12, there was a delay before they became at risk of a YCJA offense on their 12th birthday. It is therefore important to determine whether it is possible to distinguish between children whose initial cases were closed before and after they turned 12. Figure 4 shows the survival curve for three groups of adolescents, divided by age when they stopped receiving services: under 12 (risk period starting after a delay), between the ages of 12 and 14, and between the ages of 15 and 17.

It can be seen that the group of children who were under 12 at initial case closure is considerably different from the other two groups. Furthermore, the curves of the two groups aged between 12 and 17 at initial case closure are very similar, despite their ages at the start of the observation period (12–14 years or 15–17 years). It is therefore not necessary to make the distinction and they can be merged together into a single group. The YCJA incidence is 10.3% for those who were under 12 at initial case closure and 17.4% for those 12 and over at that time. More precisely, Table 2 shows how YCJA incidence changes over time, by sex and age at initial case closure.

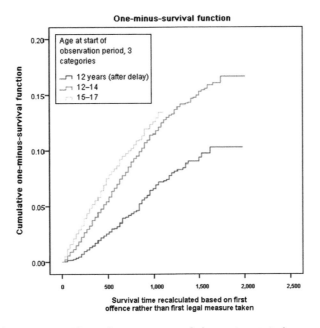

Figure 4. Cumulative YCJA incidence, by age at start of observation period.

In light of the survival curve in Figure 3 and the results in Table 2, it is clear that many more boys than girls have committed a YCJA offense. The cohort was therefore broken down into four groups based on sex and age at initial case closure. The corresponding curves are shown in Figure 5 and 5-year incidence is shown in Table 3.

Strikingly, the 5-year YCJA incidence climbs to 27.2% among boys between 12 and 17 when their initial cases were closed, compared with 14.8% for those under 12 at initial case closure. The lowest incidence is among girls whose initial cases were closed before they turned 12. Their risk is only 5.1%, compared with 7.7% for girls between 12 and 17 at initial case closure. The regression analyses below afford a better understanding of what influences this risk.

Predictors of YCJA incidence

Table 4 lists the main predictors associated with YCJA incidence among boys and girls in the cohort whose initial cases were closed before they turned 12.

Table 2. Cumulative YCJA incidence, by sex and age at initial case closure.

	Sex		Entire cohort	Age at initial case closure	
Observation period	Boys (%)	Girls (%)	Total (%)	12 and over (%)	under 12 (%)
182 days (6 months)	3.0	1.0	2.0	2.5	0.5
365 days (1 year)	6.3	2.1	4.1	5.0	1.7
730 days (2 years)	12.2	4.1	8.0	9.5	4.2
1,095 days (3 years)	17.4	6.0	11.6	13.3	7.3
1,460 days (4 years)	20.5	6.9	13.7	15.6	8.8
1,825 days (5 years)	23.4	7.1	15.4	17.4	10.3
2,006 days (5.5 years)	23.4	7.1	15.4	17.4	10.3

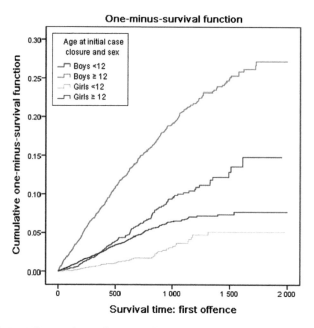

Figure 5. Cumulative YCJA incidence, by sex and age at initial case closure.

Among the boys, the only factor associated with YCJA incidence is behavioral difficulties as the grounds for the initial CPS report. More precisely, having behavioral problems more than doubles the relative risk of recurrence over the 5.5 years following initial case closure (RR = 2.3; $p < .001$). Among the girls whose cases were closed before they turned 12, as is the case with their male counterparts, having behavioral problems as a grounds for intervention more than doubles YCJA incidence (RR = 2.7; $p < .01$). The only other characteristic significantly associated with YCJA incidence among girls is CPS recurrence after initial case closure. To be more precise, girls who have one or more substantiated reports after initial case closure are at twice the risk of committing a YCJA offense (RR = 2.23; $p < .05$), than girls in this group without CPS recurrence.

Table 5 lists the main predictors of YCJA incidence among adolescents whose cases were closed when they were between the ages of 12 and 17.

Among boys, the following characteristics are associated with a *higher risk* of committing a YCJA offense: behavioral problems as grounds for intervention (RR = 2.22; $p < .001$), CPS recurrence after initial case closure (RR = 1.75; $p < .001$), more than one investigated report prior to initial postinvestigation services (RR = 1.20; $p < .001$), and court involvement at the time of initial

Table 3. Breakdown of Cohort into four groups by sex and age at initial case closure.

	Boys <12	Boys >12	Girls <12	Girls >12
n	2,057	4,640	1,663	5,892
YCJA event	141	680	40	249
Five-year incidence, YCJA offenses	14.8%	27.2%	5.1%	7.7%

Table 4. Predictors of YCJA incidence for boys and girls under 12 at initial case closure.

Characteristics of children and initial services	Boys			Girls		
	Wald	SE	RR	Wald	SE	RR
Aboriginal descent	0.41	0.51	0.72	0.14	0.74	0.76
Primary ground						
Neglect (or risk thereof)	0.18	0.29	0.89	0.41	0.63	1.50
Physical abuse (or risk thereof)	0.80	0.22	0.94	0.00	0.40	0.99
Sexual abuse (or risk thereof)	0.84	0.35	1.38	0.10	0.47	1.16
Behavioral problems	22.68***	0.18	2.31	7.47**	0.36	2.70
Abandonment	0.01	178.38	0.00	1.00	0.62	1.85
Psychological abuse	0.71	0.72	0.55	0.05	1.03	1.25
Duration of services (months)	0.82	0.01	1.00	0.10	0.01	1.00
Court involvement	1.83	0.19	0.77	0.83	0.37	1.40
Recurrence	0.64	0.18	1.15	5.90*	0.33	2.23
Discontinuity	1.43	0.17	1.23	3.00	0.35	1.84
Prior investigated reports	0.27	0.10	0.98	0.25	0.17	1.09
Global chi^2	41.10***			26.34**		

$*p < .05; **p < .01; ***p < .001.$

postinvestigation services (RR = 1.23; $p < .05$). On the other hand, initially being reported for neglect (RR = 0.65; $p < .001$) or psychological abuse (RR = 0.47; $p < .001$) appears to reduce the risk of a YCJA offense. Among the girls who were between 12 and 17 when their initial cases were closed, the following characteristics are associated with a *higher* YCJA incidence: behavioral problems as initial grounds for intervention (RR = 3.47; $p < .001$), CPS recurrence (RR = 1.83; $p < .001$), and court involvement (RR = 1.51; $p < .01$).

Discussion

The use of survival analysis techniques revealed a 15.4% YCJA incidence for the entire cohort in the 5.5 years following initial CPS case closure.

Table 5. Predictors of YCJA incidence in boys and girls aged 12 to 17 at initial case closure.

Characteristics of children and initial services	Boys			Girls		
	Wald	SE	RR	Wald	SE	RR
Age at start of observation period	3.08	0.03	1.05	0.83	0.06	0.95
Aboriginal descent	0.33	0.18	1.11	0.37	0.34	0.81
Primary ground						
Neglect (or risk thereof)	23.80***	0.09	0.65	0.20	0.14	0.94
Physical abuse (or risk thereof)	0.57	0.11	0.92	0.43	0.17	1.12
Sexual abuse (or risk thereof)	2.63	0.25	0.67	1.94	0.24	0.71
Behavioral problems	66.33***	0.10	2.22	53.90***	0.17	3.47
Abandonment	2.28	0.20	0.74	1.08	0.37	0.79
Psychological abuse	10.62***	0.23	0.47	0.90	0.31	0.72
Duration of services (months)	3.00	0.00	1.00	0.10	0.00	0.99
Court involvement	5.45*	0.08	1.23	8.26**	0.14	1.51
Recurrence	41.02***	0.09	1.75	17.75***	0.14	1.83
Discontinuity	0.87	0.08	0.98	1.45	0.13	0.86
Prior investigated reports	14.73***	0.05	1.20	0.25	0.08	1.04
Global chi^2	248.83***			105.74***		

$*p < .05; **p < .01; ***p < .001.$

Survival analyses showed that YCJA incidence is lower among children who were under 12 at initial CPS case closure than those between 12 and 17. While the 5.5-year incidence is 17.3% for those who were between 12 and 17 at initial case closure, it is only 10.3% for those not immediately at risk of committing a YCJA offense because their initial cases were closed before they turned 12. For boys, the situation is even more striking, since the risk is 14.8% among those whose initial cases were closed before they turned 12 and 27.2% for those between 12 and 17 at initial case closure.

The predictive model of YCJA incidence was tested on each of the four groups based on sex and age at initial case closure. All the factors introduced into the analysis predicted YCJA incidence better and identified a greater number of predictors for boys and girls who were 12 or older at initial CPS case closure. Two hypotheses may explain the weaker performance of the statistical models for the children who were under 12 at initial CPS case closure. First, it is possible that the smaller size of the two groups of children who were younger at initial CPS case closure might attenuate the ability of the analysis to detect relationships between the two variables (less analytical power). If that is the case, it would mean that the predictors identified in both groups are valid but that there could be others not expressed in the results due to a lack of power. Second, it is also possible that the smaller number of predictors that show up in the analyses for the children who were younger at the end of the observation period might reflect reality. Thus, the factors considered in the study seem to predict YCJA incidence for adolescents, but for younger children, other factors not considered in this study might be better determinants. The factors most likely to explain a YCJA offense may perhaps be found in the child's clinical profile and the characteristics of the home environment, which could not be considered in this study.

The most constant predictor for all four groups is initial CPS intervention for behavioral problems, which is, as specified above, specific to reasons for reporting of Quebec's system. In all the groups, behavioral problems more than double YCJA incidence (risk ratios of 2.2 to 3.5), and this effect is statistically significant in every case. Behavioral problems in childhood can thus be considered to be the first sign of potential delinquency. Although behavioral disorders have also been put forward to explain the risk of delinquency in other studies (Dandreaux & Frick, 2009; Ryan, 2012; Wright et al., 2012), the contribution of our study is to make a connection between an intervention by CPS for this reason, allowing a specific intervention concerning behavioral disorders, and the risk of YCJA incidence.

Being reported one or more times to CPS after initial case closure is also a good predictor of a later YCJA event. The strength and consistency of this effect are nonetheless more marked among those whose initial CPS cases were closed after their 12th birthday. Thus, no matter what the grounds of the initial intervention, CPS recurrence increases the risk of delinquency. Court involvement (in comparison to voluntary measures) is another factor that increases the risk of a YCJA event but only for adolescents who were between 12 and 17 at initial CPS case closure. It would be necessary to perform analyses with additional data to determine whether it is court involvement per se that increases YCJA incidence or rather the more serious psychosocial profile of cases often associated with it.

In line with the literature (Jonson-Reid & Barth, 2000b), we found the greatest number of predictors of YCJA incidence in the group of boys between ages 12 and 17 when their initial CPS cases were closed. In this group, the more investigated reports prior to receiving initial CPS postinvestigation services, the higher the YCJA incidence. A report for neglect (or risk thereof) or psychological abuse reduces YCJA incidence. It is possible that these grounds for reports were evidence of situations more clearly requiring CPS rather than a precursor to delinquency, as may be the case for a report of behavioral problems. Among those who were between the ages of 12 and 17 at initial case closure, the factors that best predict YCJA incidence are behavioral problems at the time of initial CPS intervention and repeated reports to CPS afterward. These points converge around the idea of chronic delinquency that is seen repeatedly by CPS before being dealt with under the YCJA. CPS supervision may be an opportunity to steer youths with behavioral problems away from the path to delinquency. Yet it appears that in many cases, child protective services were unable to prevent them from taking an antisocial pathway. Jonson-Reid (2002) found that "failures" of child protective services were related to children's mental health problems. Those found most strongly associated with delinquency fell into the category of serious behavioral disturbance under the YPA in Quebec. Future studies should look at the pathways of children initially reported to CPS for behavioral problems, since they are particularly at risk of committing a YCJA offense and seem to have different characteristics from those of other groups.

Yet it is important to note that, by their nature, the data available do not allow us to determine the causes of delinquency. Nevertheless, this study should be seen as a step toward research on the etiology of delinquency after initial CPS case closure. Our estimates of CPS recurrence and YCJA incidence are conservative, since the data set used in this study does not recognize a same child successively followed by different agencies. Furthermore, as it is impossible to know when children move to another region once their cases are closed, they were not censored in the calculations of relative risk of recurrence, thus underestimating the incidence. Also, using representative province-wide data enables more powerful analyses because of the sample size, and this power increases the ability to detect a relationship between two variables when there actually is such a relationship in the study population. Finally, it should be kept in mind that this study looked only at the first YCJA event occurring after children stopped receiving initial postinvestigation services. Further studies are needed to find out about adolescents repeatedly subjected to measures and sanctions under the YCJA.

Conclusion

This study sketches a preliminary portrait of YCJA incidence in Quebec after initial CPS case closure. It quantifies the scope of the phenomenon and identifies the best predictors of YCJA incidence from data available in an administrative data set that integrates CPS and YCJA services.

One of this study's biggest contributions is to document the pathway from maltreatment to delinquency among children whose CPS file was closed after a complete intervention. In our study, the most crucial predictors of delinquency are not CPS characteristics but rather behavioral problems at the time of receiving initial postinvestigation services and CPS recurrence afterward. Chronic behavioral problems (serious behavioral disturbances), severe enough to require a CPS intervention, and the fact that the youth are seen repeatedly by CPS before behavioral problems give rise to a first offense may, however, offer a worthwhile opportunity for intervention and prevention of delinquency.

Similarly, it would be interesting to investigate the importance of aspects not available in this study, such as school attendance, peer influence, and street gang membership. Another question that remains is whether estimated YCJA incidence among children under CPS supervision (15.4% after 5.5 years) differs from what might be observed in the general population. Other studies are therefore needed to assess YCJA incidence in the entire population of Quebec adolescents.

Our study only partly confirms the hypothesis that maltreatment (abuse or neglect) leads to delinquency, since behavioral problems were the only grounds associated with an extrajudicial sanction or judicial measure under the YCJA. Our findings also suggest that repeated maltreatment predisposes children to involvement in a YCJA event. It would be interesting for future studies to examine YCJA incidence with special attention to CPS recurrence. This would confirm whether the effect of CPS recurrence on YCJA incidence is due solely to chronic behavioral problems or also to other grounds for repeated intervention, such as issues of neglect or abuse.

Funding

The authors thanks Valorisation Recherche Québec and le Centre de recherche of Centre jeunesse de Montréal – Institut universitaire for their financial support.

References

Association des centres jeunesse du Québec. (2015). *Avec l'énergie du premier jour : Bilan des directeurs de la protection de la jeunesse/directeurs provinciaux 2015*. (Report No 978-2-89394-112-07) Quebec, Canada: Association des Centres jeunesse du Québec. Retrieved from http://www.cjsaglac.ca/donnees/fichiers/1/bilan-des-dpj-acjq-2015-finale_web.pdf

Baskins, D. R., & Sommers, I. (2011). Child maltreatment, placement strategies, and delinquency. *American Journal of Criminal Justice, 36*(2), 106–119.

Bender, K. (2010). Why do some maltreated youth become juvenile offenders? A call for further investigation and adaptation of youth services. *Children and Youth Services Review, 32,* 466–473. doi:10.1016/j.childyouth.2009.10.022

Bright, C. L., & Jonson-Reid, M. (2008). Onset of juvenile court involvement: Exploring gender-specific associations with maltreatment and poverty. *Children and Youth Services Review, 30,* 914–927. doi:10.1016/j.childyouth.2007.11.015. Retrieved from http://europepmc.org/arti cles/PMC2598395//reload=0;jsessionid=FVibW4TCC6Pt1oGlILxo.10

Bronfenbrenner, U. (1979). *The ecology of human development: Experiments by nature and design*. Cambridge, MA: Harvard University Press.

Case, S., & Haines, K. (2007). Offending by young people: A further risk factor analysis. *Security Journal, 20,* 96–110.

Cernkovich, S. A., Kaukinen, C. E., & Giordano, P. C. (2005). Les types de délinquantes: Une étude longitudinale des causes et des conséquences [Female offender types: A longitudinal examination of causes and consequences]. *Criminologie, 38,* 103–138.

Chiu, Y. -L., Ryan, J. P., & Herz, D. C. (2011). Allegations of maltreatment and delinquency: Does risk of juvenile arrest vary substantiation status? *Children and Youth Services Review, 33,* 855–860. doi:10.1016/j.childyouth.2010.12.007

Côté, S., Tremblay, R. E., & Vitaro, F. (2003). Le développement de l'agression physique au cours de l'enfance: Différences entre les sexes et facteurs de risque familiaux [Development of physical aggressiveness throughout childhood: Sex differences and family risk factors]. *Sociologie et sociétés, 35,* 203–220. Retrieved from http://www.erudit.org/revue/socsoc/2003/v35/n1/008517ar.pdf. doi:10.7202/008517ar

Craig, W., Petrunka, K., & Khan, S. (2011). *Better beginnings, better futures study: Delinquency trajectories of at-risk youth* (Report No PS18-1/2011E-PDF). Ontario, Canada: National Crime Prevention Center, Public Safety Canada.

Crooks, C. V., Scott, K. L., Wolfe, D. A., Chiodo, D., & Killip, S. (2007). Understanding the link between childhood maltreatment and violent delinquency: What do schools have to add? *Child Maltreatment, 12,* 269–280.

Currie, J., & Tekin, E. (2011). Understanding the cycle: Childhood maltreatment and future crime. *Journal of Human Resources, 47,* 509–549.

Dandreaux, D. M., & Frick, P. J. (2009). Developmental pathways to conduct problems: A further test of the childhood and adolescent-onset distinction. *Journal of Abnormal Child Psychology, 37*(3), 375–385.

DeGue, S., & Widom, C. S. (2009). Does out-of-home placement mediate the relationship between child maltreatment and adult criminality? *Child Maltreatment, 14*(4), 344–355.

Derzon, J. H. (2010). The correspondence of family feature with problem, aggressive, criminal, and violent behavior: A meta-analysis. *Journal of Experimental Criminology, 6*(3), 263–292.

Farrington, D. P. (1986). Early precursors of frequent offending. In J. Q. Wilson & G. C. Loury (Eds.), *From children to citizens: Families, schools, and delinquency prevention* (pp. 27–50). New York, NY: Springer.

Fitzgerald, R. (2003). *An examination of sex differences in delinquency. Canadian Centre for Justice Statistics* (Catalogue no. 85-561-MIE, No. 001). Ottawa, Canada: Statistics Canada. Retrieved from http://publications.gc.ca/collections/Collection/Statcan/85-561-MIE/85-561-MIE2003001.pdf

Ford, J. D., Hartman, J. K., Hawke, J., & Chapman, J. F. (2008). Traumatic victimization, posttraumatic stress disorder, suicidal ideation, and substance abuse risk among juvenile justice-involved youth. *Journal of Child and Adolescent Trauma, 1*(1), 75–92.

Fortin, L., & Strayer, F. F. (2000). Introduction: Caractéristiques de l'élève en troubles du comportement et contraintes sociales du contexte [Introduction: Characteristics of pupils with behavioral problems and contextual social constraints]. *Revue des sciences de l'éducation, 26,* 3–16.

Fréchette, M., & Le Blanc, M. (1987). *Délinquances et délinquants* [Deliquencies and deliquents]. Canada: Gaétan Morin.

Gatti, U., Tremblay, R., & Vitaro, F. (2009). Iatrogenic effect of juvenile justice. *Child Psychology and Psychiatry, 50*(8), 991–998.

Goodkind, S., Shook, J. J., Kim, K. H., Pohlig, R. T., & Herring, D. J. (2013). From child welfare to juvenile justice: Race, gender, and system experiences. *Youth Violence and Juvenile Justice, 11*(3), 249–272.

Hawkins, D. J., Herrenkohl, T. I., Farrington, D. P., Brewer, D., Catalano, R. F., Harachi, T. W., & Cothern, L. (2000). *Predictors of youth violence.* Washington, DC: Office of Juvenile Justice and Delinquency Prevention, US Department of Justice.

Ireland, T. O., Smith, C. A., & Thornberry, T. P. (2002). Developmental issues in the impact of child maltreatment on later delinquency and drug use. *Criminology, 40,* 359–399.

Jonson-Reid, M. (2002). Exploring the relationship between child welfare intervention and juvenile corrections involvement. *American Journal of Orthopsychiatry, 72,* 559–576.

Jonson-Reid, M., & Barth, R. P. (2000a). From maltreatment report to juvenile incarceration: The role of child welfare services. *Child Abuse and Neglect, 24,* 505–520.

Jonson-Reid, M., & Barth, R. P. (2000b). From placement to prison: The path to adolescent incarceration from child welfare supervised foster or group care. *Children and Youth Services Review, 22,* 493–516. doi:10.1016/S0190-7409(00)00100-6

Keil, V., & Price, J. M. (2006). Externalizing behavior disorders in child welfare settings: Definition, prevalence, and implications for assessment and treatment. *Children and Youth Services Review, 28*(7), 761–779.

Lanctôt, N., & Desaive, B. (2002). La nature de la prise en charge des adolescentes par la justice: Jonction des attitudes paternalistes et du profil comportemental des adolescentes [How the justice system deals with adolescent girls: At the crossroads of paternalistic attitudes and behavioral patterns]. *Déviance et Société, 26,* 463–478.

Lanctôt, N., & Le Blanc, M. (2002). Explaining adolescent females' involvement in deviance. *Crime and Justice, 29,* 113–202.

Leathers, S. J. (2006). Placement disruption and negative placement outcomes among adolescents in long-term foster-care: The role of behavior problems. *Child Abuse and Neglect, 30*(3), 307–324.

Lemmon, J. H. (2006). The effects of maltreatment recurrence and child welfare services on dimensions of delinquency. *Criminal Justice Review, 31*(1), 5–32.

Lipsey, M. W., & Derzon, J. H. (1998). Predictors of violent or serious delinquency in adolescence and early adulthood: A synthesis of longitudinal research. In R. Loeber D. P. Farrington (Eds.), *Serious and violent juvenile offenders: Risk factors and successful interventions* (pp. 86–105). Thousand Oaks, CA: Sage.

Mallett, C. A. (2014). Youthful offending and delinquency: The comorbid impact of maltreatment, mental health problems, and learning disabilities. *Child and Adolescent Social Work Journal, 31*(4), 369–392.

Maschi, T., Hatcher, S. S., Schwalbe, C. S., & Rosato, N. S. (2008). Mapping the social service pathways of youth to and through the juvenile justice system: A comprehensive review. *Children and Youth Services Review, 30*(12), 1376–1385.

Ministry of Health and Social Services. (2010). Manuel de référence sur la protection de la jeunesse [Reference Manual on Youth Protection] (Report No 10-838-04F). Québec, Canada: Gouvernement du Québec. Retrieved from http://publications.msss.gouv.qc.ca/msss/fichiers/2010/10-838-04.pdf

Moffitt, T. E., & Caspi, A. (2001). Childhood predictors differentiate life-course persistent and adolescence-limited antisocial pathways among males and females. *Development and Psychopathology, 13*, 355–375.

Moreau, J.-A. (2007). *Services sociaux et judiciaires de la naissance à la mi-adolescence: Est-il possible de prédire les trajectoires délinquantes futures?* [Social and legal services from birth to midadolescence: Can delinquent pathways be predicted?] (Master's thesis, University of Montreal, Montreal, Canada). Retrieved from https://papyrus.bib.umontreal.ca/jspui/bitstream/1866/7401/1/Moreau_Julie-Anne_2008_memoire.pdf

Newton, R. R., Litrownik, A. J., & Landsverk, J. A. (2000). Children and youth in foster care: Disentangling the relationship between problem behaviors and number of placements. *Child Abuse and Neglect, 24*(10), 1363–1374.

Pauzé, R., Toupin, J., Déry, M., Mercier, H., Cyr, M., Frappier, J.-Y., Robert, M., & Chamberland, C. (2004). *Portrait des jeunes âgés de 0–17 ans et de leur famille desservis par les Centres jeunesse du Québec, leurs parcours dans les services et leur évolution dans le temps* [Profile of children aged 17 and under and their families served by Quebec's child protective services: Their service trajectories and changes over time]. Montreal, Canada: Groupe de recherche sur les inadaptations sociales de l'enfance, Université de Sherbrooke.

Puzzanchera, C., Adams, B., & Sickmund, M. (2010). *Juvenile court statistics*. Washington, DC: Office of Juvenile Justice and Delinquency Prevention.

Ryan, J. P. (2012). Substitute care in child welfare and the risk of arrest: Does the reason for placement matter? *Child Maltreatment, 17*(2), 164–171.

Ryan, J. P., & Testa, M. F. (2005). Child maltreatment and juvenile delinquency: Investigating the role of placement and placement instability. *Children and Youth Services Review, 27*, 227–249.

Sedlak, A. J., & McPherson, K. (2010). *Survey of youth in residential placement: Youth's needs and services*. Washington, DC: Office of Juvenile Justice and Delinquency Prevention.

Shader, M. (2003). *Risk factors for delinquency: An overview*. Washington, DC: Office of Juvenile Justice and Delinquency Prevention.

Sprott, J. B., Doob, A. N., & Jenkins, J. M. (2001). Problem behaviour and delinquency in children and youth. *Juristat, 21*(4). Canadian Centre for Justice Statistics. Statistics Canada Catalogue No. 85-002-XPE. Retrieved from http://www.statcan.gc.ca/pub/85-002-x/85-002-x2001004-eng.pdf

Stewart, A., Livingston, M., & Dennison, S. (2008). Transitions and turning points: Examining the links between child maltreatment and juvenile offending. *Child Abuse and Neglect, 32*, 51–66.

Stouthamer-Loeber, M., Loeber, R., Wei, E., Farrington, D. P., & Wikström, P. H. (2002). Risk and promotive effects in the explanation of persistent serious delinquency in boys. *Journal of Consulting and Clinical Psychology, 70*(1), 111–123.

Tabachnick, B. G., & Fidell, L. S. (2013). *Using multivariates statistics* (6th ed.). Boston, MA: Pearson Education.

Tourigny, M., Mayer, M., Wright, J., Bouchard, C., Chamberland, C., Cloutier, R., & Lavergne, C. (2002). *Étude sur l'incidence et les caractéristiques des situations d'abus, de négligence, d'abandon et de troubles de comportement sérieux signalées à la Direction de la protection de la jeunesse au Québec*. Montréal, Canada: Centre de liaison sur l'intervention et la prévention psychosociales. [English summary available as *EIQ summary* (*Quebec incidence study of reported child abuse, neglect, abandonment and serious behaviour problems*), http://cwrp.ca/sites/default/files/publications/en/EIQSummary.pdf]

Tremblay, R. E. (2012). The development of physical aggression. In R. E. Tremblay, M. Boivin, & R. DeV Peters (Eds.), *Encyclopedia on early childhood development* [online]. Montreal, Canada: Centre of Excellence for Early Childhood Development and Strategic Knowledge Cluster on Early Child Development. Retrieved from http://www.child-encyclopedia.com/sites/default/files/textes-experts/en/530/the-development-of-physical-aggression.pdf

Van Wert, M., Ma, J., Lefebvre, R., & Fallon, B. (2013). An examination of delinquency in a national Canadian sample of child maltreatment-related investigations. *International Journal of Child and Adolescent Resilience, 1*(1), 48–59.

Verrecchia, P. J., Fetzer, M. D., Lemmon, J. H., & Austin, T. L. (2010). Policy implications of the effects of maltreatment type, age, recurrence, severity, and other ecological risks on persistent offending among disadvantaged boys. *Criminal Justice Policy Review, 22*, 187–218.

Widom, C. S. (2003). Understanding child maltreatment and juvenile delinquency: The research. In J. Wiig, C. S. Widom, & J. Tuell (Eds.), *Understanding child maltreatment and juvenile delinquency. From research to effective program, practice and systematic solutions.* Washington, DC: CWLA Press.

Wright, J. P., McMahon, P. M., Daly, C., & Haney, J. P. (2012). A quasi-experimental in early intervention involving collaboration between schools and the district attorney's office. *Criminology and Public Policy, 11*(2), 227–249.

Yampolskaya, S., Armstrong, M. I., & McNeish, R. (2011). Children placed in out-of-home care: Risk factors for involvement with the juvenile justice system. *Violence and Victims, 26*(2), 231–245.

Youth Protection Act. (2009). RSQ, c. P-34.1. Retrieved from http://canlii.ca/t/kncl

Youth Criminal Justice Act. (2002). S.C., c.1. Retrieved from http://laws-lois.justice.gc.ca/PDF/Y-1.5.pdf

Yun, I., Ball, J. D., & Lim, H. (2011). Disentangling the relationship between child maltreatment and violent delinquency: Using a nationally representative sample. *Journal of Interpersonal Violence, 26*(1), 88–110.

Children in Out-of-Home Care and Adult Labor-Market Attachment: A Swedish National Register Study

Torun Österberg, Björn Gustafsson, and Bo Vinnerljung

ABSTRACT

Using longitudinal national register data, we investigated labor-market attachment during the years 1993–1995 in Sweden for persons aged 25–35 years who had been in out-of-home care before the age of 18 in Sweden during the 1960s, 1970s, and 1980s. We consider whether an immigrant background has an additional influence on labor-market attachment. Compared to majority population peers, young persons who had been in foster care had shorter educations. Fewer had a strong labor-market attachment and more were dependent on social assistance. Results from multinomial regression models indicated that having been in foster care during childhood reduced the probability of high attachment to the labor-market and increased the probability of social assistance dependency, even after making adjustments for education, marital status, parenthood, domicile, and birth country. Few signs of additive effects from being both an immigrant and a former foster child are found.

A central question for social research is how education, class, and socioeconomic status in one generation affect labor-market status in the next. Do life opportunities of newborns differ based on the families they are born into, or can labor-market rewards be mainly attributed to individual choices, including efforts? While the former scenario constitutes an argument for public policies, this is not necessarily the case for the latter. In this paper we investigate the labor-market outcome for individuals who were placed in out-of-home care (foster and residential care) during childhood and/or is of foreign background.

Parents endow their children with resources (of which education is central) and affect their preferences. However, not all children grow up with two native parents. Some spend a shorter or longer period during childhood with one parent only. There is currently a large body of literature attempting to determine adult consequences of growing up in single-parent families (see section on Consequences of childhoods in foster care). In contrast, surprisingly little has been written about adult labor-market consequences of growing up with absent parents—that is, having been placed in out-of-home care (foster family and/or residential care) during childhood for a shorter or longer period of time. The situation is similar regarding research on children of ethnic backgrounds that differ from the majority and, in addition, research on children born in another country who immigrated as a child (before age 18), "child immigrants." Such persons might differ from their native-born counterparts due to a shorter exposure in the new country and due to a lower quality of parental transmission.

National register data are well suited to examine outcomes such as educational attainment and labor-market attachment. In this paper we use data from several Swedish national registers and to investigate outcomes related to labor-market attachment for individuals that have had atypical childhoods stemming from:

- having been placed in out-of-home care during childhood for shorter or longer periods (hereafter referred to as foster children, or persons having been in foster care)
- having a different ethnic background compared to the majority population—that is, having been born in another country and in addition having immigrated to the new country before age 18

A child can have experienced one or both of these states. This study aims to investigate the magnitude of the consequences of having been in out-of-home care and/or being of foreign background on the degree of labor-market attachment. We are interested in whether the sum of the effects of having met both criteria—that is, being a child immigrant and being in foster care during the formative years—are greater than the sum of the effects measured separately; that is, is there a negative additive effect? Or can we instead find a compensating effect of the double experience? We argue that it is important to study these two conditions simultaneously as many individuals experience the conditions concurrently. In the study we provide results separated for men and women.

Although atypical, the two types of childhood investigated here are not uncommon. Several national cohort studies have found between 3% and 4% of children born during the 1970s and 1980s were in care before age 18 (Vinnerljung, 1996a; Vinnerljung et al., 2007a). The fraction of individuals (all ages) born in a foreign country was about 6% in 1995. From this follows that in an average secondary school class in Sweden (consisting of around 30 pupils), one would expect to find one child who has experienced being a foster child and about two who are foreign born. Vinnerljung et al. (2008) shows, using national register data, that immigrant children are overrepresented among children in care, but after adjustments for socioeconomic background excess risks are mostly obliterated.

This paper uses unique longitudinal data and investigates labor-market status as observed for people aged 25 to 35 years for three categories of persons who were placed in out-of-home care before age 18 in Sweden during the

1960s, 1970s, and 1980s and contrasts them with majority peers without such experiences. Based on large sets of register data we describe levels of education and labor-market status measured over the 3-year period 1993 to 1995. In order to better understand how a childhood in foster care affects adult labor-market status, we control for education by estimating a multinomial logit model possessing a specification including dummies indicating former foster care and/or being of foreign background among the explanatory variables. The foster child data for this project capture labor-market attachment during the years 1993–1995, a period of severe recession in Sweden. Unemployment rose in the early 1990s and went from 1.7% in 1990 to 9.1% in 1993 (9.2% in 1994 and 8.8% in 1995). Palme et al. (2002) discusses the labor-market situation in Sweden during the 1990s. Our studied group, individual aged 25–34 years old, were however not as heavily hit by the recession as the younger age group of school leavers. It remains a task for future studies to determine whether the results reported here are valid also for other Swedish cohorts and other national contexts.

Consequences of childhoods in foster care

Examining the literature we find various studies related to our research questions. There are writings on the consequences of foster care, which in turn are related to the literature on growing up in intact families.

Research on the long-term outcomes of foster care from Europe, North America, and Australia indicate that foster care (including long-term care) seems to have at best weak compensatory long-term effects. Vinnerljung (1996b) reviewed more than 50 such studies and found that long-term outcomes for foster children (nearly regardless of measure) resembled outcomes for children who had grown up in poverty or in adverse birth homes even when the comparison group was made up of birth siblings who remained in their birth mother's care (Dumaret, 1985; Vinnerljung, 1996b). For Sweden this picture has been reinforced in a series of national cohort studies analyzing, for example, education (Vinnerljung, Öman, & Gunnarsson, 2005; Vinnerljung, Berlin, & Hjern, 2010a; Berlin, Vinnerljung, & Hjern, 2011), suicide and other avoidable mortality (Vinnerljung & Ribe, 2001; Hjern, Vinnerljung, & Lindblad, 2004; Vinnerljung et al., 2010a), hospitalization for suicide attempts and severe psychiatric illness (Vinnerljung, Hjern, & Lindblad, 2006; Vinnerljung et al., 2010, Björkenstam, Björkenstam, Ljung, Vinnerljung, & Tuvblad, 2013), teenage childbearing (Vinnerljung, Franzén, & Danielsson, 2007; Brännström, Vinnerljung, & Hjern, 2015), substance abuse (Vinnerljung et al., 2010a; von Borczykowski, Vinnerljung, & Hjern, 2013), welfare dependency (Vinnerljung et al., 2010a), Vinnerljung, Franzén, Hjern, & Lindblad, 2010), and receipt of disability pension in adulthood (Vinnerljung, Brännström, & Hjern, 2015). In a rare study on adult labor-market consequences, Cheung and Heath (1994), using data from the British National Child Development Study, found that persons with foster-care experiences had much lower levels of education, higher risks of unemployment, and if employed, were found more often in lower-level and lower-paying jobs than peers with similar educational backgrounds. Similar educational and employment outcomes in young adult ages have been found in U.S. studies (e.g., Cook, 1994; Pecora et al., 2006).

Of relevance for the transition to adulthood is that research has shown that a substantial proportion of foster children lose one or both birth parents through parental death during their time in care. At age 18, more than one of four Swedish long-term care foster children (>5 years in care) born between 1972- and 1983 had lost at least one biological parent, compared to one in 25 among normal-population peers (Franzén & Vinnerljung, 2006). Several UK and U.S. studies have also shown that only a small minority of all foster children who leave care in their late teens receive support from their foster families 1 to 2 years after care-exits. Instead, they turn to their birth families for help during the transitory years (e.g., Barth, 1990; Biehal, Clayden, Stein, & Wade, 1995; Courtney & Barth, 1996; Stein, 2006a). The results were similar to what has been found in the United Kingdom and United States (Vinnerljung, 1996b). Reasons for care entries among teenagers are a mix of behavioral problems, neglect and abuse (Vinnerljung, Sallnäs, & Kyhle-Westermark, 2001).

By being separated from their parents, foster children grow up in non-intact families. The consequences of growing up in a non-intact family are investigated in a rather large body of literature showing that children growing up in one-parent families are less successful than children growing up with two parents (Cherling, 1999). Case and associates (2000) mention several reasons concerning why divorce could have a causal effect on child outcome. It is likely that some, but not all, of those reasons also apply to foster children. Step-children and foster children may suffer from the separation per se. The child might also have lost his or her social network due to changing residential areas after the separation. Further, Case, Lin, and McLanahan (2000) have empirically tested the hypotheses that less is spent on nonbiological children than on biological children and found that in households with adoptive, stepchildren or foster children, less is spent on food, keeping household size, age, and income constant.

We are also interested in investigating whether being foreign born has an impact on labor-market attachment for former foster children. The migration to Sweden had in large been characterized by labor migration until the eighties and then moved toward a more pronounced refugee migration. Sweden was known to have low open unemployment until the early 1990s. But when the downturn hit Sweden in 1992 unemployment rose sharply. Several studies find negative wage and income gaps between immigrants and natives even when controlling for variation in educational level, for example, Gustafsson and Zheng (2006) and Hammarstedt and Shukur (2006). Some studies have focused on young adults, for example, Vilhelmsson (2002) and Behtoui (2004). Both studies indicate that after controlling for education, a foreign background constitutes a sizable labor-market disadvantage. In fact, OECD (Organisation for Economic Co-operation and Development, 2012) shows that Sweden has one of the largest gaps between native- and foreign-born persons among the rich countries. In the literature on consequences of marital disruption and growing up in a single-parent household, negative child-related effects sometimes are suggested to be related to experiences of household poverty. But this interpretation is more uncommon in studies on why young adults with immigrant background fare more poorly. Instead, theories on lack of social capital (Behtoui, 2008) and, particularly, discrimination (Rydgren, 2004) are preferred as explanatory models. Using an experimental design, Carlsson and Rooth (2007) have indeed found evidence of discrimination in the Swedish labor market.

The experience of being a foster child or a child migrant can be expected to have both common and differing impacts. Native-born foster children usually have the same first language as the majority population and do not generally differ in appearance or name and are, therefore, not expected to be discriminated against as could be the case for many child immigrants. On the other hand, after growing up, most child immigrants have biological parents who can provide networks and other kinds of support, services not available to the same extent for their native-born peers with foster child experience.

Method

Data

To be able to compare foster children's and nonfoster children's labor-market outcome we use two large register data sets: FCP (Foster Children Panel) and SWIP (the Swedish Income Panel). The FCP data consists of *all* young individuals taken into custody by the social authorities and the data originates from Statistics Sweden's register on foster children and other children the social authorities have dealt with. The register was set up at the end of the 1960s; the oldest individuals included in our data were born in 1960 and the youngest, in 1977. The observation period for labor-market outcome variables ranges from 1993 to 1995. The study uses the Swedish Income Panel (SWIP), which consists of large samples of foreign-born and Swedish-born persons who are followed over time.[1]

From the statistics Sweden Register over the Total Population (RTB) of 1978, a 1% sample of the Swedish-born population (about 77,000 individuals) and a 10% sample of the foreign-born population (about 60,000 individuals) were drawn. All individuals were observed annually until 2001. For all years from 1979 on, a 10% sample of the newly arrived immigrants were added. The source of the data is equivalent for both panels and we have information on the individual including demographic variables, educational level, and a number of variables measuring income and transfers. The population register provides annual demographic information for each person sampled, including country of birth and year of immigration. The income register derives its information from the tax authorities and also from registers of public sector transfers. Sweden has a long tradition of national registers, encompassing the entire population, with high-quality data on health and socioeconomic indicators. National registers were created and are maintained through legislation. Data originate from several sources—for example, hospital care providers, tax authorities, criminal courts, and local child welfare authorities. Reporting is legally mandatory and an individual cannot refuse to be included. Subsequently, attrition is very low for most data types (the main exception is educational attainment for immigrants).

From these two panels we have made certain subselections. In the FCP, we have outcome data for the years 1993, 1994, and 1995 but not for other years, therefore, we have restricted corresponding data from SWIP to the same years. Our main interest is to study labor-market outcomes for adults in a recession and our next selection criteria is that the individuals should be at least 25 years old in 1993. In the FCP data, the oldest individuals were born in 1960. These two restrictions mean that we will focus on individuals born between 1960 and 1968 from both data sets; the oldest observed individuals will therefore be 35 years old in 1995. Another selection criterion is having immigrated before the age of 18 so that those individuals were at risk of being taken into custody during their time in Sweden.[2]

The above delimitations give us 9,939 Swedish-born individuals that have not been foster children (based on the 1% sample from SWIP), 4,508 child immigrants that have not been foster children (based on the 10% sample from SWIP), 36,276 Swedish-born former foster children (based on the total sample from FCP) and finally 3,833 foreign-born former foster children (based on the total sample from FCP).

Dependent and independent variables

The focus for this study is on labor-market attachment in young adulthood. A high degree of attachment indicates that the person is well integrated into society and can enjoy a relatively high private consumption. Being the prototype of the dual-earner model, this is in Sweden true for men and for women. At the other extreme are people living in households with income levels that are so low that for their living expenditures they depend on social assistance. One can assume large year-to-year variation in labor-market status during single years among young adults. Therefore we use a classification of labor-market attachment that is based on personal income for the entire 3-year period: *strong labor-market attachment*—if an individual has had earnings that are three-and-a-half times the price base amount[3] at least 2 out of 3 years. This would signal that the individual is established on the labor market as an income exceeding 3.5 price base amount indicates at least a low-paying, full-time and full-year job; *unstable labor-market attachment*—if an individual has had earnings between two- and three-and-a half times the price base amount at least 2 out of 3 years; *low income*—if an individual has had earnings that are less than two times the price base amount at least 2 out of 3 years and does not belong to any of the other categories; *dependent on social assistance*—if the individual belongs to a household that has had social assistance that exceeds the amount of working income for at least 2 out of 3 years.

Since our dependent variable is a categorical one we estimate a multinominal logit model. As independent variables we will use age, dummies for educational level, a dummy variable indicating whether the individual increased his or her level of education during the period of observation (i.e., was studying), dummies for marital status including a category indicating whether the individual is cotaxed[4] with a Swedish-born person, and dummies for region of residence. In addition, we include dummies for whether the child has been a foster child— first, interacted with whether the individual is foreign-born and, second, interacted with in which region of the world the individual was born. We also separate children that entered out-of-home care for the first time before or during adolescence (age 0–12 years or age 13–17 years). Earlier research has shown that outcomes differ substantially based on whether they enter care before or during their teens (e.g., Vinnerljung, Franzén, & Danielsson, 2007; Vinnerljung & Sallnäs, 2008). The latter group is dominated by teenagers entering care due to behavioral problems (e.g., delinquency). Hereafter we will call foster children who entered care before age 13 the *FC-child-group* and those that entered care between ages 13 and 17 the *FC-teen-group*. Those who never entered care and were born in Sweden are called "the majority population" and those who never entered care but are foreign born are called "foreign born."

We report estimates for men and women separately since the effects from explanatory variables might vary by gender. We have also report on statistical interactions between having entered care with country of birth since we expect that the immigrant effect may vary between different subgroups.

Results

Educational and labor-market outcome

As discussed in the section Dependent and independent variables, we have several reasons to believe that former foster children will fare worse than the majority population as adults due to reasons such as lower endowments transmitted from parents, by other personal hardships, or by not being compensated by the transmission from the foster parents. Hence we can expect that foster children and foreign-born children will have lower educational levels than the majority (see Table 1). In the majority population, only 15% of the men and 12% of the women have elementary educations (9 years) or less. For foreign-born men and women, the corresponding figures are 20% and 22%. In contrast, about 30% of the FC-child-group and more than 40% of the FC-teen-group have only elementary schooling. The disparities between people who have experienced foster care and the majority are thus similar for men and women. Several earlier Swedish national cohort studies (Vinnerljung, Öman, & Gunnarson, 2005; Vinnerljung et al., 2010a; Vinnerljung & Hjern, 2011) have found that former child welfare clients were more likely to have only compulsory educations and that this high relative risk remained when controlling for parental characteristics (parental education and indications of parental psychopathologies) and also, most notably, for cognitive capacity (IQ; measured at time of conscription).

When turning to the other end of the scale for educational level we find a matching pattern. However, when comparing native born to foreign born who have experienced foster care, the differences are small. In other words, these results indicate that there are no negative additive effects on educational level from having experienced both immigration and foster care. In Table 1 it is also shown that former foster children are less likely to be married but more likely to be divorced (both men and women). When studying region of residence, large differences are found when comparing foreign born to native born and not when comparing foster children to nonfoster children.

In Table 2 we find that about two thirds of the majority population men have a strong labor-market attachment compared to only half of the foreign born. Among the FC-teen-group as few as around one third reach the strong labor-market attachment. These are substantial differences. Among women the share with strong labor-market attachment is generally lower. Not more than half of the majority population women have a strong labor-market attachment and only about one fourth of the female, former foster children have the equivalent economic position.

When studying the fractions of persons in households dependent on social assistance as main income source, we find large differences between those who have been in out-of-home care and those who have not. For the majority population, being dependent on social assistance is rare as only 2% belong to the category. The category with the highest fraction of "dependent on social assistance" is found among the FC-teen-group within which the proportion varies from 17% to 25%, depending on gender and whether the individual is native born or not.

Gaps in earnings among people with the same education

The labor-market attachment is weaker for the two foster care groups. We can quite safely assume that a substantial proportion of the weaker labor-market outcomes for those who have been in foster care is at least to some extent connected to the lower educational level. The register data used here is however

Table 1. Descriptive statistics for nonfoster children and foster children and for native- and foreign-born men and women.

	MEN							WOMEN						
	Majority population	foreign born	FC-child, Swedish born	FC-child, foreign born	FC-teen, Swedish born	FC-teen, foreign born	Sig.	Majority population	Foreign born	FC-child, Swedish born	FC-child, foreign born	FC-teen, Swedish born	FC-teen, foreign born	Sig.
Year of birth	1964.2	1964.1	1964.7	1964.4	1964.0	1964.2		1964.1	1964.2	1964.8	1964.8	1964.4	1964.4	
Level of education (in %)														
Elementary or less	15.2	20.4	30.3	32.3	43.7	44.2	***	12.3	22.4	29.1	30.3	43.3	44.5	***
Upper secondary 2 years	45.1	46.5	53.1	51.5	47.3	46.1	***	42.7	41.4	51.8	47.3	43.9	40.0	***
Upper secondary 3 years	12.2	11.3	7.1	5.0	3.4	3.0	***	15.8	14.0	9.5	11.9	5.1	6.7	***
Postsecondary 3 years	17.9	11.8	6.4	7.5	2.6	3.4	***	18.4	12.9	7.0	6.2	4.8	5.8	***
Postsecondary 3 years or more	7.9	5.1	1.9	2.0	0.8	0.5	***	9.2	5.8	1.8	2.7	1.4	1.3	***
Education information missing	1.7	4.9	1.2	1.7	2.3	2.8	***	1.6	3.5	0.6	1.8	1.4	1.7	***
Increased level of education during the period	5.6	5.0	2.3	1.5	1.3	1.8	***	5.5	5.5	2.8	4.1	2.7	2.0	***
Marital status (in %)							***							***
Married	23.8	26.3	16.7	19.0	15.3	20.4	***	34.2	39.2	27.0	29.0	27.2	28.7	***
Divorced	2.2	4.3	4.1	5.0	5.5	7.4	***	3.3	7.2	7.5	6.9	12.1	13.0	***
Living with Swedish born	33.7	22.4	25.5	22.9	23.0	16.8	***	46.3	30.1	38.0	29.2	34.6	24.0	***
At least one child 0–17 years	29.9	29.4	22.7	22.1	21.3	22.2	***	57.7	62.0	61.9	65.7	66.9	66.4	***
At least one child 0–3 years	24.7	22.6	18.8	18.9	15.8	15.4	***	42.2	39.8	42.3	43.4	41.5	37.5	***
County of residence:							***							***
Stockholm County	19.9	29.3	20.1	25.9	20.1	27.5	***	22.1	32.0	21.8	30.6	21.1	32.7	***
Göteborg County	9.0	10.6	11.9	12.1	10.9	10.8	***	9.1	10.5	11.4	12.0	10.2	11.4	***
Malmö County	10.0	10.5	8.5	9.1	8.0	11.7	***	9.9	10.7	8.6	9.2	8.4	10.5	***
Forest counties	20.1	9.5	18.4	9.5	20.2	8.4	***	19.9	9.8	17.9	10.8	18.6	8.3	***
Other counties	41.1	40.0	41.1	43.4	40.8	41.6		38.8	39.9	40.2	37.3	41.6	37.1	
n	4968	2216	9882	746	10513	1413		4837	2086	8186	565	6849	949	

***Indicate p value < 0.001.

Table 2. Descriptive statistics for the outcome variable: labor market attachment.

Labor market attachment	Majority population	Foreign born	FC-child Swedish born	FC-child, foreign born	FC-teen, Swedish born	FC-teen, foreign born
MEN						
Strong	67.61	50.00	50.43	38.61	34.22	28.17
Unstable	15.30	20.76	21.53	23.19	23.42	24.63
Low income	15.04	21.93	18.05	23.32	20.58	22.15
Dependent on social assistance	2.05	7.31	9.99	14.88	21.77	25.05
WOMEN						
Strong	48.42	38.35	34.49	30.8	23.74	25.61
Unstable	30.49	31.54	35.32	34.16	34.65	29.5
Low income	19.00	24.45	21.49	26.55	24.25	25.4
Dependent on social assistance	2.09	5.66	8.71	8.5	17.36	19.49

detailed and we can specify the exact educational qualification an individual has completed. We have chosen three specific educational degrees for men and three for women for which we have a sufficiently large number of observations in all groups to provide sufficient statistical power for comparing annual earnings in 1995 for individuals with the same degree. In Figure 1a men's earnings in relation to the majority population are displayed for different categories of men who completed vocational programs in metalworking, motor engineering, and woodworking together with all men are shown. Figure 1b shows results for women who completed education for domestic science, retail, clerical, and child care 2-year vocational programs and results for all women.

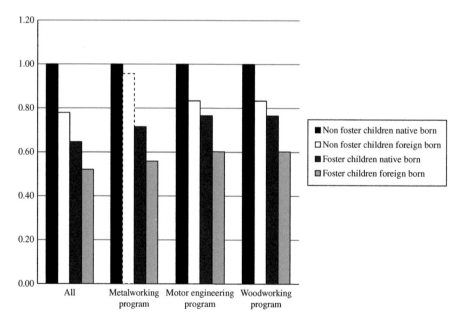

Figure 1A. Working income in 1995 in relation to native born non foster children with an equivalent educational degree – men.
Note. A dashed line indicate that the difference to a native born non foster child is insignificant p-value > 0.05. A solid line indiciate that the difference to a native born non foster child is singnificant p-value < 0.05.

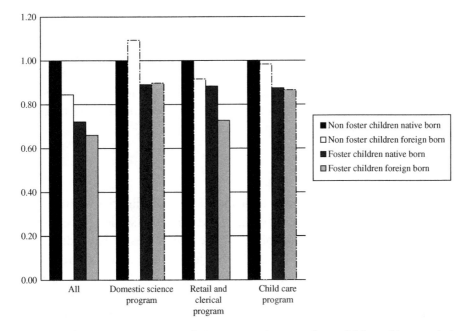

Figure 1B. Working income in 1995 in relation to native born non foster children with an equivalent educational degree – women.
Note. A dashed line indicate that the difference to a native born non foster child is insignificant *p*-value > 0.05. A solid line indiciate that the difference to a native born non foster child is singnificant *p*-value < 0.05.

We start by looking at mean annual working income in 1995 for *all* men regardless of educational qualifications. We can see that a foreign-born man earns only 78% of a majority population man's working income (Figure 1A). Those who entered foster care during childhood earn still less: 65% and 52% for a native-born man and a foreign-born man, respectively. A major source of the recorded income gap is due to differences in educational attainment. We would expect considerably smaller earnings gaps when comparing equivalent educational degrees. However, Figure 1 indicates that for male individuals this is not the case. One explanation for the large differences between natives and immigrants could be discrimination in the labor market (see section Consequences of childhoods in foster care). However, discrimination most likely cannot explain the differences between adults who have been in foster care and majority population peers, as their appearance and names are similar to those of other native-born individuals. In this case nonmeasured personal characteristics can be important, such as different forms of social exclusion mechanisms that we cannot measure with register data—for example, restricted access to facilitating labor-market contacts and low levels of support from families and other networks.

For women the picture is somewhat different. As for male individuals, the differences between majority population and former foster children and between native- and foreign-born persons are quite large in the whole sample. Foreign-born woman who also have experienced care earn only 66% of the majority population women's annual working income (134,000 SEK). However, for those with a specific educational degree, the earning gaps are smaller, though there is still a gap. Observe that among female persons, differences due to origin among those who have experienced foster care are in two out of three cases not existing.

Model estimations

We have estimated a multinomial logit model wherein differing status of labor market attachment is the dependent variable as described in section Dependent and independent variables From descriptive statistic estimations we have found rather large negative effects of having been a former foster child on the degree of labor market attachment, and there are also signs of additive effects from also being foreign born. However, foreign born persons constitute a quite heterogeneous group. More than 40% of foreign born in this study were born in the neighboring country of Finland, but there are also large groups who were born outside of Europe. To control for differences between immigrants of different backgrounds, whereby some are "visible minorities" (non-Swedish appearance; Biterman & Franzén, 2007) and some are not, we divide immigrants into eight different countries of birth groups: Sweden, Denmark or Norway, Finland, other Western countries, southern or eastern Europe, the Middle East, and other countries.

The odds-ratios from the multinomial logit model estimating labor-market outcome are shown in Table 3. The educational level has, as expected, a positive relation to a stronger labor-market attachment, being divorced has a highly negative relation, and living in Stockholm County has a positive relation.

In Figure 2A and 2B, we show the predicted probabilities from the multinomial logit estimation for different labor-market attachment based on estimates reported in Table 3 for those who never entered foster care, those who entered foster care before 13 years old, and those who entered foster care during their teens for different groups of country of birth. The predicted probabilities (Figure 2) refer to an individual born in 1964, with an upper-secondary education of 2 years, with no children, single, and living in "other counties" (Figure 2A for men and Figure 2B for women).

When we inspect labor-market attachment among those who never experienced foster care (thus controlling for education level and some demographic variables), we find quite large differences between those with a native background and those with a foreign background. For a Swedish-born man, the predicted probability of strong labor-market attachment is as high as 62% compared to 17% of a man born in the Middle East. These differences are due to either low endowment for the immigrant men (for example, that their parents do not have the connections or reputations of their native counterparts,

Table 3. Multinomial logistic regression.

Variables	Men			Women		
	2	3	4	2	3	4
Year of birth	1.035***	1.024***	0.995	1.065***	1.062***	1.046***
Reference: Swedish-born not foster child						
Swedish-born and foster child; entered care before age 13	1.586***	1.530***	4.409***	1.246***	1.310***	3.234***
Swedish-born and foster child; entered care age 13–17	2.480***	2.558***	12.191***	1.660***	1.960***	7.190***
Born in Denmark or Norway; not foster child	0.844	1.297	1.407	1.160	1.124	2.031*
Denmark or Norway foster child; entered care before age 13	1.888*	2.048*	4.278***	1.520	2.268	5.467***
Denmark or Norway foster child; entered care age 13–17	2.261***	2.523***	11.054***	1.545	1.625	5.969***
Born in Finland; not foster child	1.661***	1.133	3.004***	1.167	1.132	1.498*
Finland foster child; entered care before age 13	2.486***	1.852***	8.435***	1.421*	1.789***	3.432***
Finland foster child; entered care age 13–17	2.677***	2.692***	14.095***	1.633***	1.970***	8.869***
Born in other Western countries; not foster child	1.367	1.502*	2.851***	0.754	1.658*	1.528
Other Western countries foster child; entered care before age 13	2.124*	2.191***	5.484***	1.865	1.059	3.902*
Other Western countries foster child; entered care age 13–17	3.633***	4.519***	18.951***	1.133	1.478	3.864***
Born in southern or eastern Europe; not foster child	1.959***	2.595***	7.150***	1.006	1.106	2.766***
Southern or eastern Europe foster child; entered care before age 13 years	2.957***	4.300***	11.806***	1.249	0.985	2.308
Southern or eastern Europe foster child; entered care age 13–17	4.634***	4.322***	24.871***	1.269	1.804*	8.188***
Born in Middle East; not foster child	8.297***	7.624***	9.604***	3.527***	3.687***	3.410***
Middle East foster child; entered care before age 13	7.050***	9.536***	21.549***	5.584***	7.206***	2.602
Middle East foster child; entered care age 13–17	9.113***	7.302***	35.552***	1.852	3.530***	6.064***
Born in other countries; not foster child	2.385***	3.352***	5.114***	1.395*	2.450***	3.750***
Other countries foster child; entered care before age 13	1.559	5.022***	11.524***	0.622	2.847***	3.653*
Other countries foster child; entered care age 13–17	3.289***	2.886***	16.452***	1.296	2.242***	5.512***
Reference elementary education or less:						
Upper secondary 2 years	0.886***	0.706***	0.426***	0.699***	0.472***	0.214***
Upper secondary 3 years	0.614***	0.624***	0.135***	0.514***	0.403***	0.090***
Postsecondary less than 3 years	0.460***	0.744***	0.083***	0.326***	0.401***	0.035***
Postsecondary 3 years or more	0.222***	0.336***	0.065***	0.148***	0.134***	0.013***
No education info	1.301	1.799***	2.124***	1.196	1.742***	2.122***
Increased educational level during period	1.934***	3.899***	1.609***	1.645***	4.323***	1.841***
Reference: Single						
Married	0.945	1.127*	1.150	1.112*	1.271***	1.211*
Divorced	1.357***	1.342***	1.583***	1.418***	1.648***	2.041***
Cotaxed with Swedish born	0.721***	0.607***	0.493***	0.889*	0.848***	0.383***
Reference Stockholm County						
Göteborg County	1.452***	1.032	1.573***	1.443***	1.322***	1.709***
Malmö County	1.807***	1.229***	1.548***	1.701***	1.394***	1.480***
Forest counties	2.192***	1.232***	1.146*	2.213***	1.522***	1.497***
Other counties	1.574***	0.969	1.059	1.947***	1.481***	1.639***
Children	0.765***	0.646***	0.316***	1.789***	1.211***	1.336***
Child 0–3 years old	0.827**	0.901	0.966	1.509***	1.323***	1.082
Number of observations		29738			23472	

Dependent variable degree of labor market attachment (1 = strong attachment, 2 = unstable attachment, 3 = low income, and 4 = dependent on social assistance). A strong labor market attachment (= 1) is the comparison group. Odds-ratios presented below; figures in boldface mean that the estimate is significant on at least a 5% level.

97

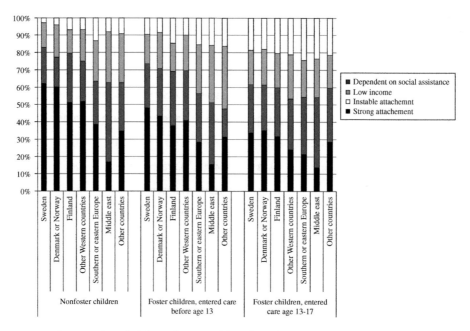

Figure 2A. Estimated probabilities from Model 3 for labor market attachment in 1993–1995. Predicted probabilities for an individual born in 1964, with short secondary education, no children, single and living in other counties – Men.

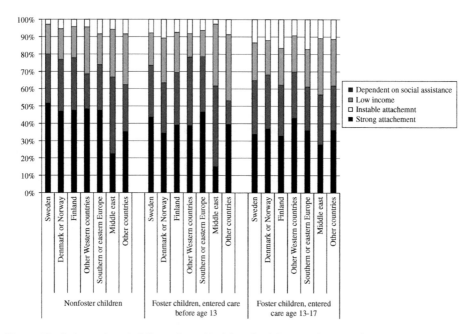

Figure 2B. Estimated probabilities from Model 3 for labor market attachment in 1993–1995. Predicted probabilities for an individual born in 1964, with short secondary education, no children, single and living in other counties – Women.

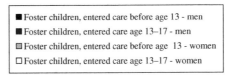

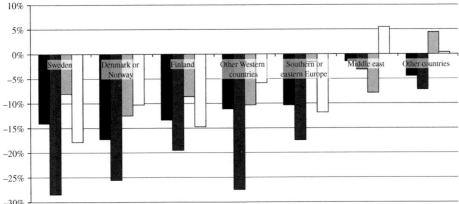

Figure 3. Within group country of birth difference between nonfoster children and the FC-child-group and nonfoster-children and the FC-teen-group in estimated percentage-point difference with a strong labor market attachment.

that immigrant men might be endowed with less Swedish-specific knowledge) or that they are discriminated against. The predictions for other categories of country of birth are in-between these extremes and the predictions for Danish or Norwegian men do not differ from a Swedish man. Turning to women the differences are smaller. Actually in several cases a foreign background does not significantly affect labor-market status (See Table 3).

In the descriptive results provided above, negative effects of having been in out-of-home care and/or being foreign born on labor-market attachment have been shown. Particularly men who entered foster care as teenagers differ considerably from the majority. In order to isolate the foster-care impact for the different countries of origin, we have calculated the percentage-point difference in estimated probabilities of labor-market attachment, the within-group differences, between those who have experienced foster care (as children or as teenagers) and those who have not, by country of birth group. In Figure 3 we show the magnitude of the "foster-care impact" holding constant the foreign-born impact. The foster-care impact is thus defined here as the difference in probability of having a particular labor-market status compared to a similar person with no experience of being a foster child but born in the same country. The predicted probabilities are derived from Table 3, thereby, allowing educational and other demographic characteristics to remain constant. From the estimates we can calculate foster-care impact for all four labor-market states but have chosen to concentrate on the state "strong labor-market attachment."

In Figure 3 it can be seen that for Swedish-born men the foster-care impact is huge. Swedish-born men who entered foster care as teenagers are estimated to be 28 percentage points less likely to have a strong labor-market attachment than those who never entered foster care. For men who entered foster care as children, the percentage-point difference is smaller but still 14 percentage points. For immigrants from the other Nordic countries or from other Western countries the foster-care impact is also large and nearly comparable in size with the effect for Swedish men. However, for immigrant men from the Middle East and "other countries," the foster-care-impact is small when calculated as the probability of strong labor-market attachment—only 1 percentage point less with a strong labor-market connection (for those who entered foster care as children) and 3 percentage points less (for those who entered foster care as teenagers) compared to those who did not experience foster care during childhood. Hence we arrive at the interesting finding for men that there are no signs of an additive effect from having been in foster care for these immigrant groups born outside of Europe.

The results for women show similar but weaker foster-care impacts (see Figure 3). A native-born woman who entered care as a teenager is estimated to be 18 percentage points less likely to have a strong labor-market attachment than a native-born woman who never entered care. For women born in the Middle East the foster-care-effect is even positive. Women who entered care as teenagers and were born in the Middle East were 5 percentage points *more* likely to have a strong labor-market attachment, compared to those who never entered care. This might be a sign of foster care having long-term compensatory effects.

Hence, for both men and women in the immigrant categories born outside of Europe, there are weak or no signs of an additive negative effect of having been in foster care during childhood regarding the outcome "strong labor-market attachment'." This could be because the hardships for these groups in the labor-market may have a mutual source and be more attributable to a lack of—or a low quality of—networks than to discrimination.

Conclusions and implications

This study based on register panel data for Sweden in the mid-90s has focused on adult outcomes for those who have experienced foster care and/or are foreign born but immigrated before 18 years of age. The results indicate that people with such atypical childhoods are as young adults on average substantially worse off compared to majority population peers. This is true with respect to educational attainment and labor-market attachment. It is also true for men as well as women. For immigrants, a background from a low- or middle-income country means a worse adult labor-market situation than being born in a high-income country. Children who enter foster care as teenagers are worse off than those who enter in younger ages. We are not aware of any previous study of the adult labor-market situation of former foster children in

Sweden. For other countries similar studies are few, and those existing have not had an opportunity to work with the kind of data we have used.

However, there are limitations in this study. Firstly, it relates only to individuals who entered care between 1960 and 1987; secondly the foreign born are those who arrived in Sweden between 1968 and 1985. Whether these results are valid also for future generation of foster children and or immigrant children is a question for future research. Further we do not know, for example, if negative outcomes are the result of the foster care experience or a result of difficulties that were present prior to the placement, hence, we cannot determine causality. Available evidence indicates that foster children and youth are a very select group from the general population (e.g., Vinnerljung & Hjern, 2014).

We also find strong negative relations in our multivariate models between former foster care experience and labor-market attachment even with controls for the lower level of education. The probable causal factors behind having been in out-of-home care or of immigrant background are numerous. There are most probably influences from the process causing the foster-care experience, most prominently the process of loss of biological parents and the child immigrant experience. Child immigrants have not been residing in the new country as long as native-born children and are, therefore, less exposed to the dominant language in the new country and have also had fewer possibilities to learn skills specific for the new country. As young adults many child immigrants are at risk of being discriminated against in the labor market based on name or appearance. Many young adults with experiences of foster care cannot count on support from their biological parents or their foster parents during the process of establishing themselves in the labor market. In this respect child immigrants are, on average, in a better position, although often less favored than the majority. For example, child migrants are likely to have access to fewer networks that are helpful in finding, obtaining and keeping a job. This might be an important reason for our findings that child immigrants from low- and middle-income countries who have been subject to foster care are not worse off than their peers with the same country of birth origin. The foster parents might have provided useful networks for finding a job.

To increase human capital among foster children (during childhood or thereafter) may be difficult although not impossible. Yet, to compensate for the lack of networks might be less demanding. In Sweden, the legal societal responsibility for the foster child ends at age 18. But those individuals who attend upper secondary school generally stay in care until they have graduated, usually at age 19. But it is now well known that parents continue to have a role in their over-18 offspring's establishment and maintenance. Höjer and Sjöblom (2010) show in an interview study that former foster children typically report a lack of support in young adulthood from birth parents but also from foster parents and from social services. For example, Fritzell and Lennartsson (2005) and Björnberg and Lätta (2007) show that financial transfers from middle-aged parents to their children over age 18 are common in Sweden. In a Canadian study, Corak and Piraino (2011) report that by age 33 as many as 40% of sons were or had been employed by the same employer as their fathers. Thus in societies in which the transition to adulthood nowadays is a much longer period than previously, setting age 18 or 19 as the end point for measures supporting foster children seems dated and calls for change. In the Swedish foster care discourse, proposals for such policies that could prolong some sort of care have been remarkably absent. This is in sharp contrast to policies in other Nordic countries and in the United Kingdom (Vinnerljung et al., 2015; Mattsson & Vinnerljung, 2016) but also to the lively debate in Sweden concerning how to overcome the labor-market disadvantages of immigrants.

Notes

1. The samples were taken from a register of the total population (RTB) kept by Statistics Sweden. This register is frequently updated and covers all persons registered as residing in Sweden. Excluded are asylum seekers waiting for a residency permit. As every person residing in Sweden has a personal number, this can be used to identify persons in various registers. It is widely believed that the register of the total population is of a high quality in many but not all respects. Undocumented immigration has not been a big issue in public debate in Sweden. However, there are reasons to believe that undocumented emigration to non-Nordic countries is underreported. This means that some (mainly foreign-born) persons registered as living in Sweden actually have left the country.
2. Further, all individuals aged 24 years or younger in 1993, who died or emigrated or immigrated during 1993 to 1995 are not included in the sample. Following a procedure used in previous studies, we have excluded persons with no registered income or transfer income during any of the 3 years (less than 1%). This group consists primarily of foreign-born individuals who have emigrated from the country without informing the Swedish authorities (and due to this measurement problem should not have been in the sample frame).
3. Price base amount (*prisbasbeloppet*) is used in Swedish legislation on for example social insurance benefits. It is linked to the consumer price index and annually updated by decision of the government. The base amount in 1995 was 35,700 SEK.
4. Two individuals are cotaxed if they are married or have at least one child in common.

References

Barth, R. (1990). On their own: The experiences of youths after foster care. *Child and Adolescent Social Work, 7*, 419–440.

Behtoui, A. (2004). Unequal opportunities for young people with immigrant backgrounds in the Swedish labour market. *Labour, 18*, 633–660.

Behtoui, A. (2008). Informal recruitment methods and disadvantage of immigrants in the Swedish labour market. *Journal of Ethnic and Migration Studies, 14*, 445–471.

Berlin, M., Vinnerljung, B., & Hjern, A. (2011). School performance in primary school and psychosocial problems in young adulthood among care leavers from long term foster care. *Children and Youth Services Review, 33*, 2489–2494.

Biehal, N., Clayden, J., Stein, M., & Wade, J. (1995). *Moving on. Young people and leaving care schemes.* London, UK: Her Majesty's Stationery Office, London.

Biterman, D., & Franzén, E. (2007). Residential segregation (Chapter 6). *International Journal of Social Welfare, 16*, 127–162.

Björkenstam, C., Björkenstam, E., Ljung, R., Vinnerljung, B., & Tuvblad, C. (2013). Suicidal behavior among delinquent former child welfare clients. *European Child and Adolescent Psychiatry, 22*(6), 349–355.

Björnberg, U., & Latta, M. (2007). The roles of the family and the welfare state – The relationship between public and private financial support in Sweden. *Current Sociology, 55*, 415–445.

Brännström, L., Vinnerljung, B., & Hjern, A. (2015). Risk factors for teenage childbirths among child welfare clients: Findings from Sweden. *Children and Youth Services Review, 53*, 44–51.

Carlsson, M., & Rooth, D.-O. (2007). Evidence of discrimination in the Swedish labor market using experimental data. *Labour Economics, 14*, 716–729.

Case, A., Lin, I.-F., & McLanahan, S. (2000). How hungry is the selfish gene? *Economic Journal, 110*(466), 781–804.

Cherling, A. J. (1999). Going to the extremes: Family structure, children's well-being and social science. *Demography, 36*, 421–428.

Cheung, Y., & Heath, A. (1994). After care: The education and occupation of adults who have been in care. *Oxford Review of Education, 20*, 361–374.

Cook, R. (1994). Are we helping foster care youth prepare for their future? *Children and Youth Services Review, 16*, 213–229.

Corak, M., & Piraino, P. (2011). The intergenerational transition of employers and earnings. *Journal of Labour Economics, 29*, 37–68.

Courtney, M., & Barth, R. (1996). Pathways of older adolescents out of foster care: implications for independent living services. *Social Work, 41*, 75–83.

Dumaret, A. (1985). IQ, scholastic performance and behaviour in sibs raised in contrasting environments. *Journal of Child Psychology and Psychiatry, 4*, 553–580.

Franzén, E., & Vinnerljung, B. (2006). Foster children as young adults: Many motherless, fatherless or orphans. A Swedish national cohort study. *Journal of Child and Family Social Work, 11*, 254–263.

Fritzell, J., & Lennartsson, C. (2005). Financial transfers between generations in Sweden. *Ageing and Society, 25*, 1–18.

Gustafsson, B., & Zheng, J. (2006). Earnings of immigrants in Sweden, 1978 to 1999. *International Migration, 44*(2), 79–117.

Hammarstedt, M., & Shukur, G. (2006). Immigrants' relative earnings in Sweden—A cohort analysis. *Labour, 20*(2), 285–323.

Hjern, A., Vinnerljung, B., & Lindblad, F. (2004). Avoidable mortality among child welfare recipients and intercountry adoptees: A national cohort study. *Journal of Epidemiology and Community Health, 58*, 412–417.

Höjer, I., & Sjöblom, Y. (2010). Young people leaving care. *Child and family social work, 15*(1), 118–127.

Mattsson, T., & Vinnerljung, B. (2016). *Åtgärder för familjehemsplacerade barn* [Legal measures to improve foster care]. Stockholm, Sweden: SNS.

Organisation for Economic Co-operation and Development. (2012). *Settling in: OECD Indicators of Immigrant Integration 2012.* Paris, France: Author.

Palme, J., Bergmark, Å., Bäckman, O., Estrada, F., Fritzell, J., Lundberg, O., Sjöberg, O., & Szebehely, M. (2002). Welfare trends in Sweden: Balancing the books for the 1990s. *Journal of European Social Policy, 12*, 329–346.

Pecora, P., Kessler, R., O'Brien, K., White, C., Williams, J., Hiripi, E., English, D., White, J., & Herrick, M.-A. (2006). Educational and employment outcomes of adults formerly placed in foster care: Results from the Northwest Foster Care Alumni Study. *Children and Youth Services Review, 28,* 1459–1481.

Rydgren, J. (2004). Mechanisms of exclusion: Ethnic discrimination in the Swedish labour market. *Journal of Ethnic and Migration Studies, 30*(4), 697–716.

Stein, M. (2006a). Young people aging out of care: The poverty of theory. *Children and Youth Services Review, 28,* 422–434.

Vilhelmsson, R. (2002). *Wages and unemployment of immigrants and natives in Sweden.* Stockholm, Sweden: Swedish Institute for Social Research Dissertation Series 56.

Vinnerljung, B. (1996a). Hur vanligt är det att ha varit fosterbarn? En deskriptiv epidemiologisk studie. *Socialvetenskaplig Tidskrift, 3*(3), 166–179.

Vinnerljung, B. (1996b). *Fosterbarn som vuxna.* Lund, Sweden: Arkiv Förlag.

Vinnerljung, B., Berlin, M., & Hjern, A. (2010a). Skolbetyg, utbildning och risker för ogynnsam utveckling hos barn [School performance, educational attainments, and risks for unfavorable development among children]. In Socialstyrelsen *Social Rapport 2010* (pp. 227–266). Stockholm, Sweden: Socialstyrelsen.

Vinnerljung, B., Brännström, L., & Hjern, A. (2015). Disability pension among adult former child welfare clients: A Swedish national cohort study. *Children and Youth Services Review, 56,* 169–176.

Vinnerljung, B., Forsman, H., Jacobsen, H., Kling, S., Kornor, H., & Lehman, S. (2015). *Översikt av kunskapsläget och exempel på genomförbara förbättringar* [Children cannot wait. A review of research on foster care with examples for viable improvements]. Stockholm, Sweden: Nordens Välfärdscenter, Projekt "Nordens barn – fokus på barn i fosterhem."

Vinnerljung, B., Franzén, E., & Danielsson, M. (2007b). Teenage parenthood among child welfare clients—a Swedish national cohort study. *Journal of Adolescence, 30,* 97–116.

Vinnerljung, B., Franzén, E., Hjern, A., & Lindblad, F. (2010b). Long term outcome of foster care: Lessons from Swedish national cohort studies. In E. Fernandez & R. Barth (Eds.), *How does foster care work? International evidence of outcomes* (pp. 206–220). London, UK: Jessica Kingsley.

Vinnerljung, B., & Hjern, A. (2011). Cognitive, educational and self-support outcomes of long-term foster care versus adoption. A Swedish national cohort study. *Children and Youth Services Review, 33,* 1902–1910.

Vinnerljung, B., & Hjern, A. (2014). Consumption of psychotropic drugs among adults who were in societal care during their childhood. *Nordic Journal of Psychiatry, 68,* 611–619.

Vinnerljung, B., Hjern, A., & Lindblad, F. (2006). Suicide attempts and severe psychiatric morbidity among former child welfare clients—a national cohort study. *Journal of Child Psychology and Psychiatry, 47,* 723–733.

Vinnerljung, B., Hjern, A., Ringbäck Weitoft, G., Franzén, E., & Estrada, F. (2007a). Children and young people at risk. Social Report 2006. *International Journal of Social Welfare, 16*(Suppl. 1), S163–S202.

Vinnerljung, B., Öman, M., & Gunnarson, T. (2005). Educational attainments of former child welfare clients—a Swedish national cohort study. *International Journal of Social Welfare, 14,* 265–276.

Vinnerljung, B., & Ribe, M. (2001). Mortality after care among young adult foster children in Sweden. *International Journal of Social Welfare, 10*(3), 164–173.

Vinnerljung, B., & Sallnäs, M. (2008). Into adulthood: A follow-up study of 718 youths who were placed in out-of-home care during their teens. *Journal of Child and Family Social Work, 13,* 144–155.

Vinnerljung, B., Sallnäs, M., & Kyhle Westermark, P. (2001). *Sammanbrott i tonårsplaceringar* [Breakdowns in placements of teenagers in out-of-home care]. Stockholm, Sweden: Socialstyrelsen.

von Borczykowski, A., Vinnerljung, B., & Hjern, A. (2013). Alcohol and drug abuse among young adults who grew up in substitute care—findings from a Swedish national cohort study. *Children and Youth Services Review, 35,* 1954–1961.

The Relationship Between Child Maltreatment, Intimate Partner Violence Exposure, and Academic Performance

Lisa R. Kiesel, Kristine N. Piescher, and Jeffrey L. Edleson

ABSTRACT
This article presents a longitudinal examination of the association between children's experiences of child maltreatment (CM) and intimate partner violence (IPV), alone and in combination, with children's academic performance. Integrated, administrative data from the Minnesota Departments of Education and Human Services were used to obtain a sample of 2,914 children. Data provided an opportunity to study comparisons of single (CM or IPV) and combined experiences (CM-IPV), longitudinally observe the impact of these experiences on academic functioning, and make comparisons to the general population. Results revealed significant differences in school attendance and math and reading performance by adverse experience. Children exposed to CM and IPV, individually or in combination, underperformed at school. IPV-exposed children had the poorest outcomes. Findings highlight the need for dedicated screening for adverse childhood experiences, particularly IPV exposure, and devoting greater educational and social service resources as a means of promoting future school achievement and adult functioning.

Children's experiences of child maltreatment (CM) and exposure to parental intimate partner violence (IPV) often co-occur. A recent national study found that over half (56.8%) of children in the United States who reported being exposed to IPV had also been maltreated in their lifetimes (Hamby, Finkelhor, Turner, & Ormrod, 2010). However, estimates of the prevalence of child exposure to IPV in the United States vary. IPV exposure has been estimated to affect three- to four-million children annually (Yates, Dodds, Sroufe, & Egeland, 2003). Retrospective studies indicate that 20%–37% of adults report having witnessed IPV in their families, and the total number of children in the United States exposed to IPV has been estimated at 17.8 million (Overlein, 2010).

Researchers have examined the impact of CM and IPV exposure on child adjustment over the past three decades. This body of work has progressed from examining the frequency and intensity of single adverse events to considering the co-occurrence and effects of experiencing multiple adverse events, or polyvictimization. Findings of this research have been used to shape policy and practice in child welfare and other related fields. For example, research on the co-occurrence of CM and IPV exposure has led to the creation of policies that support increased domestic violence training for child welfare professionals and that articulate child welfare responses to cases alleging child exposure to domestic violence (Edleson & Malik, 2008; Schechter & Edleson, 1999). At the same time, the field of child welfare has been influenced by policies that require child welfare professionals to attend to issues of child well-being more broadly than safety and permanency alone (U.S. Department of Health and Human Services [US DHHS], n.d.). A better understanding of how commonly occurring adverse experiences (i.e., CM and IPV exposure) affect key aspects of child well-being, including the educational well-being of children, is needed to assist the field in better supporting children's well-being. With this in mind, the current study was developed to explore the effects of CM and IPV exposure on children's academic performance over time.

Child maltreatment, intimate partner violence, and child outcomes

Multiple studies and reviews have revealed negative associations between children's exposure to CM and IPV and children's social, emotional, and behavioral adjustment; health; mental health; and school performance (Evans, Davies, & DiLillo, 2008; Kitzmann, Gaylord, Holt, & Kenny, 2003; Trickett & McBride-Chang, 1995; Wolfe, Crooks, Lee, McIntyre-Smith, & Jaffe, 2003). IPV exposure through witnessing the violence, hearing about it later, or living in the aftermath of the violence has been found to have adverse effects on child development (Holden, 2003). Exposure to IPV as a child is highly associated with an increased risk of IPV victimization or perpetration in adulthood (Ehrensaft et al., 2003; Whitfield, Anda, Dube, & Felitti, 2003; Widom, Czaja, & Dutton, 2014), and both CM and IPV experiences are associated with other social and career difficulties in later life (Currie & Widom, 2010; Fergusson & Horwood, 1998; Paradis et al., 2009; Silvern et al., 1995).

Adverse childhood experiences (ACEs)

More recently, long-term negative outcomes of experiencing multiple childhood adversities have been identified by researchers using the ten-item Adverse Childhood Experiences Scale (*Adverse Childhood Experiences Questionnaire: Finding your ACE score*, 2006). Childhood physical, sexual, and emotional abuse, neglect, and the abuse of one's mother constitute five of 10 adverse childhood experiences (ACEs) associated with negative outcomes both during and well beyond childhood. ACEs are associated with learning and behavior problems (Burke, Hellman, Scott, Weems, & Carrion, 2011), risky behaviors, and increased suicide attempts in adolescence and adulthood (Anda et al., 2002; Dube et al., 2001); ACEs also predict lifelong difficulties that are (independently) associated with poor mental and physical health outcomes (Dube et al., 2003; Shonkoff et al., 2011). Negative developmental outcomes accumulate as the types of adverse experiences increase (Felitti et al., 1998; Graham-Bermann & Seng, 2005). However, less attention has been paid to understanding the impact of combined adverse experiences on children's academic performance—a pivotal indicator of success for children that has long-lasting implications for adult functioning.

School performance, academic achievement, and ACEs

CM and IPV exposure are core facets of the ACE scale. Experiencing CM and being exposed to IPV have been associated with poor school performance and academic achievement. These associations hold whether the adverse experiences are studied independently or as co-occurring issues; however, much less is known about these outcomes when experiences co-occur.

CM is predictive of children's success at school. Maltreatment has been associated with reduced attendance and increased student mobility (Eckenrode, Rowe, Laird, & Brathwaite, 1995; Leiter & Johnsen, 1994). Research has shown that maltreated children move twice as often as their nonmaltreated peers during their school years (Eckenrode et al., 1995) and demonstrate low levels of achievement—significantly lower levels than those of their nonmaltreated peers (Berger, Cancian, Han, Noyes, & Rios-Salas, 2015; Piescher, Colburn, Hong, & LaLiberte, 2014; Smithgall, Gladden, Howard, Goerge, & Courtney, 2004). Impaired academic performance, evidenced by eligibility for special education, grade retention, and lower grades have also been observed among maltreated children (Romano, Babchishin, Marquis, & Fréchette, 2015). Physically abused children have shown increased disciplinary problems and grade retention and fare poorly on academic achievement and social-emotional development assessments (Coohey, Renner, Hua, Zhang, & Whitney, 2011; Eckenrode, Laird, & Doris, 1995; Kurtz, Gaudin, Howing, & Wodarski, 1993; Kurtz, Gaudin, Wodarski, & Howing, 1993). Moreover, children who have been neglected demonstrate the poorest academic achievement and are at the greatest risk for school failure (De Bellis, Hooper, Spratt, & Woolley, 2009; Fantuzzo, Perlman, & Dobbins, 2011).

Children's IPV exposure and its effects over time appear to also impact academic performance. IPV exposure has been associated with diminished cognitive development and academic performance. For example, Artz, Jackson, Rossiter, Nijdam-Jones, Géczy, and Porteous (2014), in their comprehensive review of the impact of child IPV exposure, found children to have lower reading scores, greater speech and language impairment, poorer academic progress or performance, and greater academic failure than those of their nonexposed peers.

Koenen, Moffitt, Caspi, Taylor, and Purcell (2003) found that IPV exposure suppressed children's IQ scores, even when controlling for both genetic differences (twin study) and the trauma of child maltreatment. Studies by Huth-Bocks and colleagues (Huth-Bocks, Levendosky, & Semel, 2001) and Graham-Bermann and colleagues (Graham-Bermann, Howell, Miller, Kwek, & Lilly, 2010) found that exposure to IPV was directly and indirectly associated with preschool children's poorer verbal abilities, and Thompson and Whimper (2010) found that among early adolescents, having been exposed to IPV was a unique predictor of low reading level. Finally, a study in Sri Lanka demonstrated an association between those currently experiencing exposure to IPV at home and both poor school attendance (less than 80%) and low achievement (failing at or below the 40th percentile) (Jayasinghe, Jayawardena, & Perera, 2009).

While the understanding of the academic effects of CM and IPV exposure on children is growing, less information about the combined effects of co-occurring CM and IPV on children's academic functioning is available. This is due, in part, to the difficulty of gathering and integrating these sensitive data, as our service systems are splintered and services for CM and IPV are often handled by different entities that exist outside of the educational system. However, research has demonstrated that children who experience multiple childhood adversities fare poorly academically, including exhibiting learning problems and lower achievement (Burke et al., 2011; Holt, Finkelhor, & Kantor, 2007). Understanding the impact of multiple adversities on education is also complicated by the way these impacts influence one another and interact over time, and by the interaction with the functioning of systems surrounding the child (Artz et al., 2014; Romano et al., 2015). Huang and Mossige (2012) studied students in their final year of secondary school and found that experiences of violence, both singular and multiple types, negatively affect child educational outcomes—directly and indirectly—by impacting children's social-emotional health. These findings suggest that research on the impact of multiple, co-occurring types of childhood adversities is needed before opportunities for intervention can most clearly be identified.

Current study

Our study examined the association between children's experiences of CM and IPV (alone and in combination) with academic performance over time. Specifically, our longitudinal investigation explored the association of children's CM experience, IPV exposure alone, and co-occurring CM and IPV exposure (CM-IPV), with children's school attendance and academic achievement. Examining the impact of multiple adverse experiences on children's academic performance and achievement is in alignment with recent child welfare efforts to address child well-being from a more holistic perspective. Current federal evaluations of state-level child and family services include three areas of well-being outside of child safety and permanency: (a) increasing family capacity to meet their children's needs, (b) children receiving needed services to meet their educational needs, and (c) receipt of adequate mental and physical health services (US DHHS, n.d.). The U.S. Administration on Children, Youth and Families (ACYF) recently provided more-specific guidance for public child welfare agencies on the promotion of child well-being, including cognitive functioning as a central aspect of well-being that includes language skills, problem solving and decision making skills, academic achievement, and school engagement and attachment (US DHHS, 2012). Thus, developing mechanisms to aid our understanding of the relationship between adverse experiences, including CM and IPV, and academic outcomes are of particular importance to the field of child welfare.

Our study relied on integrated, secondary, administrative data from multiple sources within the Minnesota Departments of Education and Human Services. Our study overcame one of the major difficulties previously mentioned—namely, accessing and integrating splintered data on children's exposure and their academic performance. Utilizing data reported from July 2005 through June 2009, this study provided an opportunity to study comparisons of single (CM or IPV) and combined occurrences (CM-IPV), observe the impact of these experiences on academic functioning over multiple years, and make comparisons to the general population via a four-group design. The purpose of this study was to explore the impact over time of children's exposure to IPV and CM on child school attendance and academic performance. The central research question of this study was, Did the experience of single and/or multiple childhood adversities (CM only, CM+ IPV, IPV only) differentially affect children's school attendance and academic achievement?

Method

This study relied upon integrated secondary data from the Minnesota-Linking Information for Kids (Minn-LInK) project—a project that utilizes statewide administrative data from multiple agencies, including the Minnesota Departments of Human Services (DHS) and Education (DOE), to answer questions about the effects of policies, programs, and practice on the well-being of children in Minnesota. For this study, data from DHS and DOE were used in accordance with data sharing agreements between the Minn-LInK project at the University of Minnesota and these state agencies. Data-sharing agreements allowed the use of identified data for the purpose of conducting research on families and children. The university's institutional review board approved the use of these secondary data for these purposes, and all identifiers were removed from the data file once cross-system matching was achieved (de-identification).

The existence of the Minn-LInK project allowed study researchers to overcome some of the aforementioned challenges regarding splintered systems (and therefore splintered data) by providing established processes and protocols to (a) acquire administrative data for research purposes, (b) store and utilize sensitive data while ensuring data confidentiality and security, and (c) effectively integrate data across systems that do not share child-level, unique identifiers. However, policy and practice research has rarely been the primary focus of administrative data collection. While this reality does not prohibit the successful design, implementation, and completion of research, it does present researchers with unique challenges related to study design and time frames for study group selection that occur after the data has been collected. Instances in which data system conditions drove the structure of this study have been noted in this article.

Sampling procedures

Four groups were created based on children's experiences of child maltreatment and intimate partner violence: child maltreatment alone (CM), exposure to intimate partner violence alone (IPV), child maltreatment and IPV exposure (CM-IPV), and a general population comparison group (GP). Child protection records were initially used to determine whether children would be eligible for inclusion in one of the CM, IPV, or CM-IPV groups or in the GP comparison group. First, child protection records were used to select children (aged 7 – 13 years) whose *first experience* of alleged child maltreatment, either abuse or neglect, was substantiated in a child protection investigation that occurred between July 2005 and June 2006 (Year 1). The age range was chosen to correspond to the timing of academic testing to provide longitudinal data for three time points and to control for timing of CM; testing began at grade 3 and continued annually through grade 8, with reading given again in grade 10 and math given in grade 11.

Records of children who experienced substantiated CM were split into two group—CM and CM-IPV—based on an indicator of intimate partner violence included in a Structured Decision Making (SDM) risk assessment that was conducted during the child protection investigation (Children's Research Center, 2008). SDM is one required component of screening completed by child protection workers based on their knowledge of a family's history and circumstances, as ascertained by interviews with and assessments of all family members. Family Risk Assessments, a component of SDM, are completed during a child protection assessment to determine whether or not a family should be referred for ongoing case management and again prior to ending case management services to document elimination of safety concerns and risk reduction for ongoing maltreatment. SDM data can be linked to other administrative data through the Minn-LInK project to obtain a fuller picture of the families and children who undergo assessments.

The CM group included children with substantiated maltreatment but whose caregiver(s) did *not* report experiencing current involvement in a harmful relationship as a victim of domestic violence. It should be noted that in Minnesota child exposure to domestic violence (abuse or neglect) is not assessed as child maltreatment but assessed as a risk factor. Initial Identification of IPV exposure was made using SDM data only in Year 1. In response to the SDM prompt "Primary caregiver involved in harmful relationships," the response "Yes, as the victim of domestic violence" was recorded as YES to IPV; all other responses were recorded as NO. Domestic violence was defined as "adult mistreatment of one another and evidenced by hitting, slapping, yelling, berating, verbal/physical abuse, physical fighting (with or without injury), continuing threats, ultimatums, intimidation, frequent separation/reconcilia-tion, involvement of law enforcement and/or domestic violence programs, restraining orders, or criminal reports" (Minnesota Department of Human Services, 2012, p. 16).

The CM-IPV group was then composed of children with substantiated maltreatment for whom at least one caregiver also reported current involvement in a harmful relationship as a victim of domestic violence.

Next, child protection records were used to select children for the IPV group. Children (aged 7–13 years) whose *first experience* of alleged child maltreatment remained unsubstantiated in a child protection investigation occurring in Year 1 but whose child protection record indicated at least one caregiver reporting current involvement in a harmful relationship as a victim of domestic violence (based on Year 1 SDM Risk Assessment data) were included in this group. For all CM, CM-IPV, and IPV groups, children whose caregiver (s) reported prior or subsequent IPV outside of Year 1 were excluded. History of IPV exposure was determined by SDM data prompt "Caregiver(s) have a history of domestic violence" (Yes or No) in Year 1, and subsequent IPV exposure between July 2006 and June 2009 determined through any subsequent collection of SDM data with the prompt "Caregiver(s) has experienced domestic violence since last risk assessment" (Yes or No).

Utilizing Link Plus, probabilistic record linkage software that is part of the Registry Plus suite of tools made available by the Centers for Disease Control (Centers for Disease Control and Prevention, 2010), child protection data for children in the CM, CM-IPV, and IPV groups were linked to their respective education data for years 2 (AY2006-2007) through 4 (AY2008-2009). A matched general population (GP group) comparison sample was then drawn from statewide education records using propensity score matching methods. Propensity score matching is a method for the pairing of treatment and control units with similar propensity scores, while unmatched units are all discarded (Rosenbaum, 1989; Rosenbaum & Rubin, 1983). The method of matching for this study was stratification on the propensity score (Rosenbaum & Rubin, 1984). Children (aged 7–13 years) who were not involved in an accepted case of child maltreatment prior to or during the study period (July 2005–June 2009) were eligible for inclusion in the GP group. The GP group was matched to the population of children included in the CM, CM-IPV, and IPV groups based upon gender, race, an indicator of family income (eligibility for free or reduced-price lunch), grade, and school.

It is important to note that children with a first child maltreatment report preceding July 2005 and those who did not have continuous education records (i.e., those who moved out of state or attended home school) throughout the study period (July 2005 – June 2009) were excluded and not eligible for inclusion in any study group. Additionally, children who qualified for special education services prior to the 2005 – 2006 school year were excluded to allow us to test the relationship between maltreatment and special education entry although this analysis is not included here. The 2005 – 2006 academic year was chosen for sample development as it coincided with the implementation of the Minnesota Comprehensive Assessment-II and allowed for a large sample of repeated measures of academic performance across a 3-year observation period. The Minnesota Comprehensive Assessment was changed in 2011, therefore prohibiting repeated measures in years outside of the study timeframe. Children who experienced subsequent substantiated child maltreatment ($n = 269$) and those whose caregivers reported subsequent IPV ($n = 62$) were removed from groups to maintain the integrity of the grouping variable; the GP group was similarly adjusted. The final sample totaled 2,914 children (see Table 1 for breakdown by group). The sample included slightly more females than males. The majority of children were White; although approximately one fourth were Black; American Indian, Asian/Pacific Islander, and Hispanic children were also represented in the sample (generally representative of Minnesota child protection population; Children and Family Services, 2008) though in smaller proportions. For the total population, 81% (2,224) qualified for free or reduced-price lunch. Children were distributed fairly evenly across grades in the sample in Year 1 (see Table 2).

Measures

Demographic indicators

All demographic indicators for the current study were derived from Minnesota Department of Education records. Demographic indicators included gender (male, female), Year 1 grade level (2, 3, 4, 5, 6, 7, 8), race/ethnicity (American Indian/Alaskan Native, Asian/Pacific Islander, Hispanic, Black, White), and an indicator of family income. For this study, a child's eligibility for free and reduced-price school lunch due to family income eligibility requirements was used as a proxy for family income. Eligibility was coded for each child based on whether or not they were eligible for free or reduced-price lunches (a binary variable). Eligibility was determined using Year 2 education records, coinciding with the first year of academic performance measurement.

Table 1. Demographic characteristics of study sample ($N = 2,914$).

Group	Description	Free or Reduced-Price Lunch % (n)	Race/Ethnicity % (n)					Gender % (n)	
			American Indian/ Alaskan Native	Asian/Pacific Islander	Hispanic	Black	White	Male	Female
CM (n = 1,062)	Substantiated CM without IPV	78.6 (776)	6.7 (71)	3.5 (37)	9.5 (101)	27.3 (264)	55.5 (589)	40.0 (425)	60.0 (637)
CM-IPV (n = 264)	Substantiated CM with IPV	87.6 (218)	10.6 (28)	4.5 (12)	11.7 (31)	24.9 (72)	45.8 (121)	48.5 (128)	51.5 (136)
IPV (n = 131)	Unsubstantiated CM with IPV	86.3 (107)	14.5 (19)	4.6 (6)	6.9 (9)	25.2 (33)	48.9 (64)	43.5 (57)	57.0 (74)
GP (n = 1,457)	No CM investigation; IPV unknown	81.9 (1123)	7.5 (110)	3.7 (54)	9.1 (132)	23.3 (339)	55.4 (822)	43.0 (626)	57.0 (831)
Total (n = 2,914)		80.7 (2224)	7.8 (228)	3.7 (109)	9.4 (273)	24.3 (708)	54.8 (1236)	42.4 (1236)	57.6 (1678)

Note. CM = substantiated child maltreatment; IPV = intimate partner violence, GP = general population comparison.

Table 2. Sample by grade in year 1 ($N = 2,914$).

				Grade			
	2	3	4	5	6	7	8
%	17.3	17.7	13.2	12.3	12.6	12.7	14.2
(n)	(503)	(516)	(384)	(359)	(368)	(370)	(414)

School attendance

A yearly attendance rate for each child was calculated for Years 2–4. The rate was calculated by summing the average daily attendance (ADA) for grades, schools, or districts in a given year and dividing it by that child's average daily "membership" or enrollment at a school (ADM) for the year. The attendance ratio could range from .01 (very low, or almost no attendance) to 1.0 (perfect attendance). Use of this ratio as opposed to another measure of attendance allowed for comparisons of children across school districts whose school year lengths vary in Minnesota. Rates of missing data were 5% (Year 2), 8.6% (Year 3), and 11.0% (Year 4). Significant differences in missing data among groups as measured through chi-square analysis were not evident.

Reading and Math achievement

Minnesota children are mandated to complete standardized math and reading tests (Minnesota Comprehensive Assessments) in grades 3–8, reading tests in grade 10, and math tests in grade 11. The use of scale scores (Years 2–4) allowed for comparisons over time as they are adjusted to reflect performance at each grade level, reflect the percentile rank of each student (0–99). Scores above 50 represented proficiency and met No Child Left Behind (NCLB) federal school policy standards ([DOE], 2011). Rates of missing reading data were 22.8% (Year 2), 26.1% (Year 3), and 39.0% (Year 4). Statistically significant differences in missing data among groups as measured through chi-square analysis were not evident with the exception of Year 3, in which fewer GP group scores were missing. Rates of missing math data were 29.8% (Year 2), 38.9% (Year 3), and 41.5% (Year 4). Statistically significant differences in missing data among groups as measured through chi-square analysis were not evident. Missing data may in part be accounted for by student absences on testing days and lack of reading testing in grades 9 and 11 and math testing in grades 9 and 10.

Data analyses

All data were analyzed using SPSS Statistics, version 23.0; data supported a longitudinal model using a 3-year study period (based upon the academic calendar [July to June], 2006–2007, 2007–2008, and 2008–2009). Given the large sample size and homogeneity of the data, despite non-normative data distribution, ANOVA with post hoc pairwise contrasts were used to assess mean differences in outcomes between groups at the three annual testing points for attendance rate and for reading and math scale scores. The Generalized Estimating Equation (GEE) procedure using gamma probability distribution was used as a measure of changes in outcomes between groups over time (Liang & Zeger, 1986). GEE with continuous variable response was administered for all outcomes of interest. In other words, GEE was used to determine whether the CM, CM-IPV, IPV, and GP groups' outcomes were changing at different rates over the 3-year investigation period. The more typical application of mixed MANOVA for a repeat measures longitudinal design was not possible due to violation of test assumptions, including normality and sphericity.

Results

School attendance

Mean attendance rates in Year 2 were relatively high, with all groups demonstrating greater than 90% mean attendance. A one-way, between-subjects ANOVA revealed statistically significant differences among group mean attendance rates for all 3 years (Year 2 $F(3, 2750) = 24.971, p < .001$); (Year 3 $F(3, 2660) = 15.453, p < .001$); (Year 4 $F(3, 2590) = 17.220, p < .001$). Post hoc comparisons using the Tukey HSD test indicated the higher mean attendance rate of the GP group was statistically significant compared to those of all other groups across all time periods (Table 3).

Attendance trajectories decreased for all groups during the study time period, with the CM, CM-IPV, and IPV groups' mean attendance falling below 90% by Year 3 (Figure 1). A longitudinal analysis using GEE was conducted to assess whether the change trajectories in annual school attendance rates over 3 years

Table 3. Average attendance rates and reading and math scale scores.

	Year 2		Year 3		Year 4	
	M	SD	M	SD	M	SD
Attendance						
CM	0.92	0.09	0.91	0.12	0.90	0.14
CM-IPV	0.92	0.09	0.91	0.11	0.90	0.12
IPV	0.90	0.09	0.90	0.11	0.89	0.01
GP	0.94	0.06	0.93	0.08	0.93	0.09
Reading						
CM	49.64	14.86	49.64	12.87	49.30	12.54
CM-IPV	48.35	13.75	47.24	12.99	48.43	12.11
IPV	45.82	15.74	45.21	11.70	47.16	10.75
GP	52.95	14.80	52.90	13.53	52.75	13.10
Math						
CM	47.09	13.98	45.70	13.55	42.81	14.56
CM-IPV	44.98	13.29	42.58	13.81	43.19	15.59
IPV	43.71	13.50	42.09	14.19	39.19	14.80
GP	51.04	13.91	50.00	14.43	47.29	16.17

Note. CM = substantiated child maltreatment, IPV = intimate partner violence, GP = general population comparison.

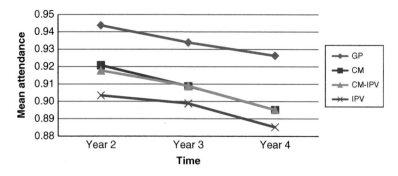

Figure 1. Annual attendance rates over 3 years.

significantly differed among the CM, CM-IPV, IPV, and GP groups. Significant differences in the rates of change between groups across time were found (QIC = 142.024, Wald $\chi2$ = 81.386, $p < .001$; see Table 4 for group parameter estimates). An examination of pair-wise contrasts indicated statistically significant differences between the CM, CM-IPV, and IPV groups compared to the GP group across time periods (Table 5). Though differences existed between CM, CM-IPV, and IPV subgroups, they were not statistically significant.

School achievement

As seen in Table 3, mean reading and math scores were moderate; on average, the only group to meet NCLB standards over time was the GP group for reading. A one-way, between-subjects ANOVA revealed statistically significant differences among group mean achievement rates for all 3 years: Reading (Year 2 $F(3, 2247) = 15.096$, $p < .001$); (Year 3 $F(3, 2149) = 22.002$, $p < .001$);

Table 4. Generalized estimating equation (GEE) parameter estimates.

Group		β	SE	95% Wald Confidence Interval Lower	Upper
Attendance					
	CM	− .026	.0035	− .033	− .019
	CM-IPV	− .029	.0058	− .040	− .017
	IVP	− .038	.0087	− .056	− .021
	GP	− .058	.0074	− .073	− .044
Reading					
	CM	− .064	.0107	− .085	− .043
	CM-IPV	− .079	.0180	− .114	− .044
	IPV	− .116	.0251	− .165	− .067
	GP	3.772	.0245	3.724	3.820
Math					
	CM	− .090	.0127	− .115	− .065
	CM-IPV	− .132	.0222	− .176	− .089
	IPV	− .174	.0306	− .234	− .114
	GP	4.075	.0168	4.042	4.107

Note. CM = substantiated child maltreatment, IPV = intimate partner violence, GP = general population comparison.

Table 5. Analysis of group grand means, standard deviations, and pairwise contrasts for attendance ($n = 8{,}007$ observations), and reading ($n = 6{,}181$) and Math ($n = 5{,}532$) achievement over 3 years.

Outcome	Mean	SD	Contrasts	Mean difference	P value
Attendance	0.92	0.10	GP vs. CM	0.02***	<.001
			GP vs. CM-IPV	0.03***	<.001
			GP vs. IPV	0.04***	<.001
Reading	50.95	13.81	GP vs. CM	3.33***	<.001
			GP vs. CM-IPV	4.90***	<.001
			GP vs. IPV	6.90***	<.001
			CM vs. IPV	3.57*	<.05
Math	47.13	14.75	GP vs. CM	4.21***	<.001
			GP vs. CM-IPV	6.93***	<.001
			GP vs. IPV	7.70***	<.001
			CM vs. IPV	3.49*	<.05

Note. CM = substantiated child maltreatment, IPV = intimate partner violence, GP = general population comparison. Standardized tests of achievement were administered in grades 3–8 only; thus the full sample was not included in assessing differences in reading and math achievement.

(Year 4 $F(3, 1773) = 13.896, p < .001$); Math (Year 2 $F(3, 2043) = 21.533, p < .001$); (Year 3 $F(3, 1776) = 24.197, p < .001$); (Year 4 $F(3, 1701) = 14.436, p < .001$). Post hoc comparisons using the Tukey HSD test indicated that the higher mean reading score for the GP group was statistically significant compared to all other groups across all time periods and that in Year 3 the lower IPV group mean score was statistically significant compared to the CM group (Table 3). Post hoc comparisons using the Tukey HSD test indicated that the higher mean math score for the GP group was statistically significant compared to all other groups across all time periods and that in Year 3 the CM-IPV group mean score was significantly lower than that of the CM group.

Longitudinal analyses, again using GEE, were conducted to assess differences between each group's academic achievement as measured by MCA-II reading and math scores over 3 years. Statistically significant differences between groups across time were found for both reading (QIC = 617.731, Wald $\chi^2 = 58.305$, $p < .001$) and math achievement (QIC = 849.654, Wald $\chi^2 = 87.833, p < .001$; see Table 4 for parameter estimates). The trajectories for children in each group are shown in Figures 2 and 3 below.

An examination of pair-wise contrasts indicated that for both reading and math, for the CM, CM-IPV, and IPV groups the difference in the rates of change were statistically significant compared to the GP and that the CM and IPV groups' rates of change differed statistically from one another (see Table 5).

Attempts were made to improve the GEE models for both attendance and achievement, adding covariates including grade, sex, SES, and maltreatment type. Using this same GEE procedure to examine attendance rate and academic achievement differences over time, the models were statistically significant overall, with both higher grade level and low SES associated with lower rates of attendance and achievement. However, these models were not as good a fit as

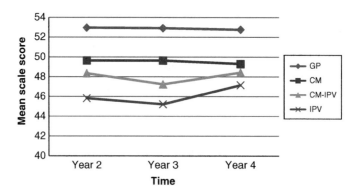

Figure 2. Reading scale scores over 3 years.

looking at group effects alone, as indicated by higher goodness-of-fit measures, and are thus not presented in the current article.

Discussion

We used integrated, longitudinal, administrative data from two child-serving systems to understand the associations between adverse childhood experiences —namely, child maltreatment and IPV exposure—and school attendance and academic achievement. Differences due to type of adverse experience were explored and proved significant in predicting children's academic outcomes. Thus, it appears that there is a clear relationship between these adverse experiences and children's school attendance and academic performance. This relationship is supported by previous research on both CM (e.g., Piescher et al., 2014; Smithgall et al., 2004) and IPV exposure (Graham-Bermann et al., 2010; Koenen et al., 2003; Thompson & Whimper, 2010). These academic outcomes represent only the first 3 years post CM and IPV exposures; we can only speculate upon the potential trajectory set by early academic challenges for long-term outcomes.

Children who experienced CM and/or were exposed to IPV—whether alone or in combination—attended school at significantly lower rates than their peers who had no history of child protection service involvement. Interestingly, the

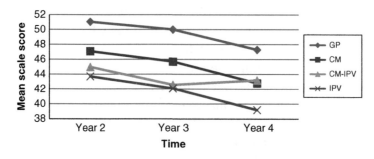

Figure 3. Math scale scores over 3 years.

attendance of the IPV group was the lowest overall. Evidence consistent with an increased negative effect of the combined experience of CM and IPV on academic performance (as has been found in earlier studies; see Felitti et al., 1998; Hughes, Parkinson, & Vargo, 1989) was not demonstrated in this study. Although some outcomes demonstrated that combined exposure to IPV and CM was associated with similar problematic outcomes (i.e., attendance) compared to CM exposure alone, children exposed only to IPV consistently exhibited the lowest attendance and achievement levels. While there were some demonstrated associations of combined CM-IPV and poor negative outcomes, there appeared to be also a possible "protective" association for IPV-exposed children when CM also occurred.

It is beyond the capacity of our study to determine the process by which the IPV group finds itself at greatest disadvantage in the outcomes; however, the role of service intervention (particularly child protective services [CPS] intervention) possibly played a part in these discrepant outcomes. Though the CM, CM-IPV, and IPV groups were all CPS-involved due to allegations of child maltreatment, maltreatment allegations of the IPV group were determined to be unsubstantiated. The CM and CM-IPV groups, however, were determined to have substantiated child maltreatment, thus mandating (in the vast majority of cases) further CPS response and intervention. CPS interventions, which targeted the adverse experiences under study, if successful, would have changed the adversities children were facing (i.e., stopped the maltreatment from continuing). In addition, the very interventions offered through CPS, such as individual and family therapy, may have helped children in the CM and CM-IPV groups with their social, emotional, and behavioral adjustment and, thus, assisted them in achieving better academic performance.

All groups of children with adverse experiences of child maltreatment and/or IPV exposure—whether alone or in combination—performed significantly worse than the matched general population group (who were never CPS involved) on standardized reading and math achievement tests. Although the IPV group fared consistently the worst across both reading and math achievement, it is important to note that *all* children who experienced the adversities of child maltreatment and/or IPV exposure struggled to demonstrate proficiency on standardized tests of achievement; the matched comparison group also struggled to demonstrate proficiency but not to the same extent as adversity-exposed groups. In comparison, the Minnesota Department of Education reported that in 2009 (Year 3 of this study) the proportion of students proficient in reading ranged from 78% in grade 3 to the lowest percentage at 65% in grade 7; the proportion of students proficient in math scores in that same year ranged from 79% in grade 3 to 41% in grade 11 (next lowest was 58% in grade 8) (Minnesota Department of Education, n.d.). Findings of this study support the proposition that in addition to the adverse experiences of CM and IPV exposure themselves, proficiency (or lack thereof) may also be associated with other unmeasured variables that are associated with risk characteristics of the groups studied (e.g., low income, housing instability, parental chemical and mental health issues). Conversely, other protective factors present within IPV families may also play a role. It remains unknown whether protective capacities of IPV families differed from those of the CM or CM-IPV families and thus played a role in these differential outcomes.

Several authors argue that the stress of severe domestic violence suppresses children's academic achievement (see Koenen et al., 2003) or that school absences caused by staying home to protect mothers may account for poorer academic achievement (Cunningham & Baker, 2004). The degree of social service intervention may also play a part in these differences. Groups exposed to CM and CM-IPV included only children substantiated for CM, thus further child protection system response was likely mandated. IPV cases, however, may not have been mandated for further care. It is perhaps this loss of intervention that differentiates these children from the others in achievement trajectories. This is not to argue that a child protection intervention is necessary but that perhaps children exposed only to IPV should more consistently receive community-based service interventions of some kind (Cross, Mathews, Tonmyr, Scott, & Ouimet, 2012; Edleson, 2006). Further research may seek to explore more specifically the role of child protection or other intervention in the outcomes of children exposed to IPV.

Study limitations

Conducting secondary analyses of administrative data, as stated earlier, gives rise to several limitations. These data were not collected for the purpose of our research; variables may not be consistently answered for each case or always answered in the same way. An effort has been made to interpret the data as accurately as possible given these limitations. However, it remains that we relied on three particular measures to describe children's academic performance—namely, attendance and achievement on Minnesota standardized tests of math and reading. Other measures, such as grade retention, GPA, and disciplinary involvement may provide corroborative or different conclusions about children's academic performance.

The sample is subject to the limits of administrative data, as well as the limits of self-disclosure of IPV to the child protection authority for the SDM risk assessment. Additionally, the matched general population comparison group was drawn from the full population of grades 2–8 in the Minnesota education database. The authors selected children for the comparison group who were not involved in an accepted case of child maltreatment in Minnesota; thus, the extent of child maltreatment in the comparison group is assumed to be marginal. However, no measures of IPV exposure existed outside of the child protection records for the full population. Therefore the actual rates of IPV exposure in the comparison group is unknown. Thus, it is unknown how our study sample may skew differences between children who experience the adversities of child maltreatment and IPV exposure as compared to their peers.

Characteristics of the data limited the range of statistical analyses available. GEE procedures were utilized in place of MANOVA due to test assumption violation. This alternative for longitudinal analysis provides means testing but does not provide an indication of the magnitude of differences.

Implications

Research

Integrating secondary data for ethical research on vulnerable populations can be a daunting task. Although studies using integrated, administrative data rely on case matching and secondary data analysis techniques, these studies often take a great deal of resource investment. Developing relationships with data owners, creating legal documents for data sharing, integrating data across systems, and understanding the nature and the strengths and limitations of the data are all time-consuming tasks. Yet, this research can lead to valuable information about children and families served by our local and state systems. In addition, because the indicators (i.e., variables) used for our research come directly from the child- or family-serving systems themselves, findings can be more easily translated into practice while necessary changes to data collection that were identified in the research can be made. Successful models of data sharing and integration are necessary for on-going research on child well-being. While some models exist, replication of these projects is necessary to continue to advance the edge of knowledge and inform policy and practice at local, national, and international levels. Successful replication will require that persons working on existing projects provide assistance to newly developing projects as well as network with other extant projects to allow for efficient and effective use of administrative data. In addition, funding for these endeavors (whether private or public) is critically important for development, enhancement, and ongoing project costs.

While using secondary data from multiple sources is not without its challenges and limitations, continued investigation into the association between children's adverse experiences and their functioning in other domains, such as in schools, should be undertaken. This research should combine both primary and secondary data collection to better understand these phenomena. Research to better understand differential service provision to children and families served by the Child Protection System is warranted. For example, what services are provided for families who report IPV but whose child maltreatment allegations go unsubstantiated? Investigating potential mediating and moderating effects of service provision on the association between exposure and academic outcomes is also necessary to develop an array of services that meet the needs of children and families. In addition, much more work needs to be undertaken to disentangle the effects of compound or repeated exposure to CM and/or IPV on children's academic outcomes. While CM and IPV exposure can be detrimental experiences for youth, they are not uncommon (e.g., Hamby, Finkelhor, Turner, & Ormrod, 2010). A better understanding of these issues is of utmost importance. More specifically examining the pathways from CM and IPV to specific outcomes, examining more closely the interactions of impacts, such as school achievement with other impacts, may also help pinpoint potential points of intervention to change the trajectories of children exposed to adverse experiences.

Practice and policy

Although the goals of safety and permanency for children continue as critically important mandates in child protection, the field has witnessed an increased focus on child well-being in recent years (Mason, 2012; US DHHS, 2012). This focus was partly driven by concern that even when children were protected from harm and were in a permanent and stable home, a large number of children who had come to the attention of CPS were not doing well across many domains of functioning, raising questions about their overall well-being. The field must develop a shared understanding of the role of CPS in supporting child well-being before further progress can be made. At present, evaluation of states' child welfare programs (via the Child and Family Service Review) includes a focus on well-being (including educational well-being) for only those children who are placed out-of-home (e.g., in foster care; US DHHS, 2014). The practice of promoting child well-being ought to apply at minimum to all children and families who have come to the attention of child protection services. In addition to expanding the groups of children to whom the well-being outcomes apply, well-being requires both greater specificity to allow measurement of progress and specific guidance on how to improve this indicator. As it stands, each state, and in some states each county, independently interprets these outcomes. Consistency and accountability for well-being outcomes is not possible with such divergent definitions.

Our data point to the need for early intervention with children experiencing both CM and IPV exposure. The impacts of these exposures could be reduced through earlier identification of ACEs among children and the provision of evidence-based intervention, such as trauma-informed care, and improvements in cross-system integration. When a child comes to the attention of professionals for either CM or exposure to IPV, close attention should be paid to what else is going on in that child's life and home. Further, in response to the common co-occurrence of CM and IPV, there is a need to seek greater integration of both child and adult care systems and educational institutions. While local child protection services may choose to exceed these requirements and provide additional services to family members, it is left to the individual agencies to make these decisions. There is no such mandate for services within educational systems. This may leave service provision uneven across cases.

Better assessment of child needs is required when adults receive intervention for IPV, and the same is true for adults' needs when children receive intervention for CM. Strengthening connections between and the capacity of the systems around the child, such as family, school, and community services, may increase protection against the risk of negative long-term outcomes.

Conclusion

Our data indicate that children exposed to both CM and IPV, individually or in combination, underperform at school. In particular, IPV-exposed children appear to have the poorest outcomes, which calls for dedicated attention to their needs. Many state policies dictate services to be provided to victims of maltreatment. Screening for ACEs, particularly IPV exposure, and devoting greater educational and social service resources to supporting these children may help them recover from the effects of these adversities and set a more positive course for their future school achievement and adult functioning.

Funding

This research was supported by funds from the Canadian Institutes of Health Research (CIHR) Institute of Gender and Health (IGH) and Institute of Neurosciences Mental Health and Addictions (INMHA) to PreVAiL (Centre for Research Development in Gender, Mental Health and Violence across the Lifespan). This research was carried out via the Minnesota Linking Information for Kids (Minn-LInK) project, made possible by collaborative partnership between the Minnesota Department of Human Services, Minnesota Department of Education, and the University of Minnesota's School of Social Work.

References

Adverse childhood experiences questionnaire: Finding your ACE score. (2006). National Council of Juvenile and Family Court Judges. Retrieved from http://www.ncjfcj.org/sites/default/files/Finding%20Your%20ACE%20Score.pdf

Anda, R. F., Chapman, D. P., Felitti, V. J., Edwards, V., Williamson, D. F., & Croft, J. B. (2002). Adverse childhood experiences and risk of paternity in teen pregnancy. *Obstetrics and Gynecology, 100*(1), 37–45.

Artz, S., Jackson, M. A., Rossiter, K. R., Nijdam-Jones, A., Géczy, I., & Porteous, S. (2014). A comprehensive review of the literature on the impact of exposure to intimate partner violence on children and youth. *International Journal of Child, Youth and Family Studies, 5*(4), 493–587.

Berger, L. M., Cancian, M., Han, E., Noyes, J., & Rios-Salas, V. (2015). Children's academic achievement and foster care. *Pediatrics, 135*(1), e109–e116.

Burke, N. J., Hellman, J. L., Scott, B. G., Weems, C. F., & Carrion, V. G. (2011). The impact of adverse childhood experiences on an urban pediatric population. *Child Abuse and Neglect, 35*(6), 408–413.

Centers for Disease Control and Prevention (CDC). (2010). *Registry Plus, a suite of publicly available software programs for collecting and processing cancer registry data.* Atlanta, GA: U.S. Department of Health and Human Services, Centers for Disease Control and Prevention, National Center for Chronic Disease Prevention and Health Promotion. Retrieved from http://www.cdc.gov/cancer/npcr/

Children and Family Services. (2008). *Minnesota's child welfare report, 2007: Report to the 2008 Minnesota legislature.* Retrieved from https://edocs.dhs.state.mn.us/lfserver/Legacy/DHS-5408-ENG

Children's Research Center. (2008). *The structured decision making® model: An evidence-based approach to human services.* National Center for Crime and Delinquency. Retrieved from http://www.nccdglobal.org/sites/default/files/publication_pdf/2008_sdm_book.pdf

Coohey, C., Renner, L. M., Hua, L., Zhang, Y. J., & Whitney, S. D. (2011). Academic achievement despite child maltreatment: A longitudinal study. *Child Abuse and Neglect, 35*, 688–699.

Cross, T. P., Mathews, B., Tonmyr, L., Scott, D., & Ouimet, C. (2012). Child welfare policy and practice on children's exposure to domestic violence. *Child Abuse and Neglect, 36*, 210–216.

Cunningham, A., & Baker, L. (2004). *What about me! Seeking to understand a child's view of domestic violence.* London, Canada: Centre for Children and Families in the Justice System. Retrieved from http://www.lfcc.on.ca/what_about_me.pdf

Currie, J., & Widom, C. S. (2010). Long term consequence of child abuse and neglect on adult economic well-being. *Child Maltreatment, 15*(2), 111–120.

De Bellis, M. D., Hooper, S. R., Spratt, E. G., & Woolley, D. P. (2009). Neuropsychological findings in childhood neglect and their relationships to pediatric PTSD. *Journal of the International Neuropsychology Society, 15*, 868–878.

Dube, S. R., Anda, R. F., Felitti, V. J., Chapman, D. P., Williamson, D. F., & Giles, W. H. (2001). Childhood abuse, household dysfunction, and the risk of attempted suicide throughout the life span: Findings from the Adverse Childhood Experiences Study. *Journal of the American Medical Association, 286*(24), 3089–3096.

Dube, S. R., Felitti, V. J., Dong, M., Chapman, D. P., Giles, W. H., & Anda, R. F. (2003). Childhood abuse, neglect and household dysfunction and the risk of illicit drug use: The adverse childhood experiences study. *Pediatrics, 111*(3), 564–572.

Eckenrode, J., Laird, M., & Doris, J. (1993). School performance and disciplinary problems among abused and neglected children. *Developmental Psychology, 29*(1), 53–62.

Eckenrode, J., Rowe, E., Laird, M., & Brathwaite, J. (1995). Mobility as a mediator of the effects of child maltreatment on academic performance. *Child Development, 66*, 1130–1142.

Edleson, J. L. (2006). A response system for children exposed to domestic violence: Public policy in support of best practices. In M. Feerick & G. B. Silverman (Eds.), *Children exposed to violence* (pp. 191–211). Baltimore, MD: Brookes.

Edleson, J. L. & Malik, N. (2008). Collaborating for family safety: Results from the greenbook multi-site evaluation (special issue). *Journal of Interpersonal Violence, 23*(7), 871–875.

Ehrensaft, M. K., Cohen, P., Brown, J., Smailes, E., Chen, H., & Johnson, J. G. (2003). Intergenerational transmission of partner violence: A 20-year prospective study. *Journal of Consulting and Clinical Psychology, 71*(4), 741–753.

Evans, S. E., Davies, C., & DiLillo, D. (2008). Exposure to domestic violence: A meta-analysis of child and adolescent outcomes. *Aggression and Violent Behavior, 13*, 131–140.

Fantuzzo, J. W., Perlman, S. M., & Dobbins, E. K. (2011). Types and timing of child maltreatment and early school success: A population-based investigation. *Children and Youth Services Review, 33*(8), 1404–1411.

Fergusson, D. M., & Horwood, L. J. (1998). Exposure to interparental violence in childhood and psychosocial adjustment in young adulthood. *Child Abuse and Neglect, 22*(5), 339–357.

Felitti, V. J., Anda, R. F., Nordenberg, D., Williamson, D. F., Spitz, A. M., Edwards, V., Koss, M. P., & Marks, J. S. (1998). Relationship of childhood abuse and household dysfunction to many of the leading causes of death in adults: The Adverse Childhood Experiences (ACE) Study. *American Journal of Preventive Medicine, 14*, 245–258.

Graham-Bermann, S. A., Howell, K. H., Miller, L. E., Kwek, J., & Lilly, M. M. (2010). Traumatic events and maternal education as predictors of verbal ability for preschool children exposed to intimate partner violence (IPV). *Journal of Family Violence, 25*, 383–392.

Graham-Bermann, S. A., & Seng, J. (2005). Violence exposure and traumatic stress symptoms as additional predictors of health problems in high-risk children. *Journal of Pediatrics, 146*, 349–354.

Hamby, S., Finkelhor, D., Turner, H., & Ormrod, R. (2010). The overlap of witnessing partner violence with child maltreatment and other victimizations in a nationally representative survey of youth. *Child Abuse and Neglect, 34*, 734–741.

Holden, G. W. (2003). Children exposed to domestic violence and child abuse: Terminology and taxonomy. *Clinical Child and Family Psychology Review, 6*(3), 151–160.

Holt, M. K., Finkelhor, D., & Kantor, G. K. (2007). Multiple vicitimization experiences of urban elementary school students: Associations with psychosocial functioning and academic performance. *Child Abuse and Neglect, 31*(5), 503–515.

Huang, L., & Mossige, S. (2012). Academic achievement in Norwegian secondary schools: The impact of violence during childhood. *Social Psychology of Education, 15*(2), 147–164.

Hughes, H. M., Parkinson, D., & Vargo, M. (1989). Witnessing spouse abuse and experiencing physical abuse: A "double whammy"? *Journal of Family Violence, 4*, 197–209.

Huth-Bocks, A. C., Levendosky, A. A., & Semel, M. A. (2001). The direct and indirect effects of domestic violence on young children's intellectual functioning. *Journal of Family Violence, 16*(3), 269–290.

Jayasinghe, S., Jayawardena, P., & Perera, H. (2009). Influence of intimate partner violence on behaviour, psychological status and school performance of children in Sri Lanka. *Journal of Family Studies, 15*, 271–283.

Kitzmann, K. M., Gaylord, N. K., Holt, A. R., & Kenny, E. D. (2003). Child witnesses to domestic violence: A meta-analytic review. *Journal of Consulting and Clinical Psychology, 71*(2), 339–352.

Koenen, K. C., Moffitt, T. E., Caspi, A., Taylor, A., & Purcell, S. (2003). Domestic violence is associated with environmental suppression of IQ in young children. *Development and Psychopathology, 15*, 297–311.

Kurtz, P. D., Gaudin, J. M., Jr., Howing, P. T., & Wodarski, J. S. (1993). The consequences of physical abuse and neglect on the school aged child: Mediating factors. *Children and Youth Services Review, 15*, 85–104.

Kurtz, P. D., Gaudin, J. M., Jr., Wodarski, J. S., & Howing, P. T. (1993). Maltreatment and the school-aged child: School performance consequences. *Child Abuse and Neglect, 17*, 581–589.

Leiter, J., & Johnsen, M. C. (1994). Child maltreatment and school performance. *American Journal of Education, 102*(2), 154–189.

Liang, K. Y., & Zeger, S. L. (1986). Longitudinal data analysis using generalized linear models. *Biometrika, 73*, 13–22.

Mason, S. (2012). Child well-being as a federal priority in child welfare. *Families in Society: Journal of Contemporary Social Services, 93*(3), 155–156.

Minnesota Department of Education. (n.d.). *A common sense plea to avoid the Minnesota math test massacre.* Retrieved from http://www.swsc.org/cms/lib04/MN01000693/Centricity/

Domain/124/A%20Common%20Sens%20Plea%20to%20Avoid%20the%20Minnesota%20Math%20Test%20Massacre.pdf

Minnesota Department of Human Services. (2012). *The Structured Decision Making system for Child Protective Services: Policy and procedures manual.* Retrieved from http://nrccps.org/wp-content/uploads/minnesota-sdm-policy-and-procedures-manual-052012.pdf

Overlein, C. (2010). Children exposed to domestic violence: Conclusions from the literature and challenges ahead. *Journal of Social Work, 10*(1), 80–97.

Paradis, A. D., Reinherz, H. Z., Giaconia, R. M., Beardslee, W. R., Ward, K., & Fitzmaurice, G. M. (2009). Long-term impact of family arguments and physical violence on adult functioning at age 30 years: Findings from the Simmons Longitudinal Study. *Journal of the American Academy of Child and Adolescent Psychiatry, 48,* 290–298.

Piescher, K., Colburne, G., Hong, S., & LaLiberte, T. (2014). Child protective services and the achievement gap. *Children and Youth Services Review, 47,* 408–415. doi:10.1016/j.childyouth.2014.11.004

Romano, E., Babchishin, L., Marquis, R., & Fréchette, S. (2015). Childhood maltreatment and educational outcomes. *Trauma, Violence, and Abuse, 16*(4), 418–437.

Rosenbaum, P. R. (1989). Optimal matching for observational studies. *Journal of the American Statistical Association, 84*(408), 1024–1032.

Rosenbaum, P. A., & Rubin, D. B. (1983). The central role of the propensity score in observational studies for causal effects. *Biometrika, 70*(1), 41–55.

Rosenbaum, P. R., & Rubin, D. B. (1984). Reducing bias in observational studies using subclassification on the propensity score. *Journal of the American Statistical Association, 79,* 516–524.

Schechter, S., & Edleson, J. L. (1999). *Effective intervention in domestic violence and child maltreatment: Guidelines for policy and practice.* Reno, NV: National Council of Juvenile and Family Court Judges.

Shonkoff, J. P., Garner, A. S., Siegel, B. S., Dobbins, M. I., Earls, M. F., McGuinn, L., Pascoe, J., & Wood, D. L. (2012). The lifelong effects of early childhood adversity and toxic stress. *Pediatrics, 129*(1), 232–246.

Silvern, L., Karyl, J., Waelde, L., Hodges, W. F., Starek, J., Heidt, E., & Min, K. (1995). Retrospective reports of parental partner abuse: Relationships to depression, trauma symptoms and self-esteem among college students. *Journal of Family Violence, 10,* 177–202.

Smithgall, C., Gladden, R. M., Howard, E., Goerge, R., & Courtney, M. (2004). *Educational experiences of children in out-of-home care.* Chicago, IL: Chapin Hall at the University of Chicago.

Thompson, R., & Whimper, L. A. (2010). Exposure to family violence and reading level of early adolescents. *Journal of Aggression, Maltreatment and Trauma, 19*(7), 721–733.

Trickett, P. K., & McBride-Chang, C. (1995). The developmental impact of different forms of child abuse and neglect. *Developmental Review, 15,* 311–337.

U.S. Department of Health and Human Services, Administration for Children and Families, Administration on Children, Youth, and Families, Children's Bureau. (2012). *Promoting social and emotional well-being for children and youth receiving child welfare services.* Information memorandum (#ACYF-CB-IM 12–04). Retrieved from https://www.acf.hhs.gov/programs/cb/resource/im1204

U.S. Department of Health and Human Services. (n.d.). *Child and Family Services Reviews quick reference items list.* Administration on Children, Youth, and Families. Retrieved from http://www.acf.hhs.gov/sites/default/files/cb/cfsr_quick_reference_list.pdf

U.S. Department of Health and Human Services. (2014). *Child and Family Services Review procedures manual—Round 3.* Administration on Children, Youth, and Families, Children's Bureau. Retrieved from http://www.acf.hhs.gov/sites/default/files/cb/round3_procedures_manual.pdf

Whitfield, C. L., Anda, R. F., Dube, S. R., & Felitti, V. J. (2003). Violent childhood experiences and the risk of intimate partner violence in adults: Assessment in a large health maintenance organization. *Journal of Interpersonal Violence, 18,* 166–185.

Widom, C. S., Czaja, W., & Dutton, M. A. (2014). Child abuse and neglect and intimate partner violence victimization and perpetration: A prospective investigation. *Child Abuse and Neglect, 38*(4), 650–663.

Wolfe, D. A., Crooks, C. V., Lee, V., McIntyre-Smith, A., & Jaffe, P. G. (2003). The effects of children's exposure to domestic violence: A meta-analysis and critique. *Clinical Childhood Family Psychology Review, 6*(3), 171–187.

Yates, R. M., Dodds, M. F., Sroufe, L. A., & Egeland, B. (2003). Exposure to partner violence and child behavior problems: A prospective study controlling for child physical abuse and neglect, child cognitive ability, socioeconomic status, and life stress. *Development and Psychopathology, 15*, 199–218.

Index

Note: Page numbers in *italics* refer to figures
Page numbers in **bold** refer to tables

INDEX

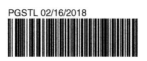